About the author

Kitty Campion, leading author... care and trained medical herbalist, is a member of the British Herbal Medical Association and associate member of the British Holistic Medical Association. She has received considerable recognition through her books and the medical centre that she runs; her recent books: *Kitty Campion's Vegetarian Encyclopaedia, Kitty Campion's Handbook of Herbal Health* and *Kitty Little's Book of Herbal Beauty*, have brought her name to public attention and proved to many that alternative remedies are often the most effective. She stands as the best advertisement for her own theories. She is a fervent believer in helping people to take responsibility for their own health care, grows her own herbs and travels the world in search of fresh information. She was recently awarded a PhD by the American School of Natural Healing.

Author's note

Herbs are very potent healing tools. Misused they can be harmful. If you are ill or have the slightest doubt about the direction of your own health care you need to work with a competent qualified naturopath well-versed in nutritional therapy and the medicinal use of herbs. The advice offered in this book is general, not specific, and the author can only take responsibility for people she has personally met, examined and agreed to work with.

Also published by Century Hutchinson:

Kitty Campion's Vegetarian Encyclopaedia (1986)

A WOMAN'S HERBAL

Kitty Campion

CENTURY
London Melbourne Auckland Johannesburg

First published in 1987 by Century Hutchinson Ltd
Brookmount House, 62–65 Chandos Place, Covent Garden,
London WC2N 4NW

Century Hutchinson Australia Pty Ltd
PO Box 496
16–22 Church Street
Hawthorn
Victoria 3122
Australia

Century Hutchinson New Zealand Limited
PO Box 40-086
Glenfield
Auckland 10
New Zealand

Century Hutchinson South Africa (Pty) Ltd
PO Box 337
Bergvlei
2012 South Africa

Photoset in Linotron Sabon by
Rowland Phototypesetting Ltd
Bury St Edmunds, Suffolk
Printed and bound in Great Britain by
Richard Clay Ltd, Bungay, Suffolk

Reprinted 1987, 1988

British Library Cataloguing in Publication Data
Campion, Kitty
    A woman's herbal: how to use herbs
    for head to toe beauty as well as body
    detoxification, stress reduction and
    aging gracefully.
    1. Beauty, Personal 2. Herbs
    I. Title
    646.7′2   RA778
    ISBN 0-7126-1635-7

Illustrations of herbs taken from
John Parkinson's *Paradisus* (1629)

Contents

Dedication

If I had but one wish it would be to live in a world like this one, at a time like the present, with friends like the ones I am blessed with now: Ruth, Chris, Liz and Ayşe who love me through the grieving times as well as through the good.

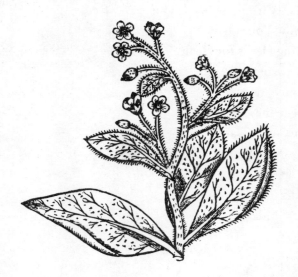

Introduction

There is an inherent bliss in being female in which I revel. It is something which a distressing number of the women I meet have lost sight of. Some because they are bogged down in a morass of being somebody's wife or mother, others finding it excruciating to be a sex symbol when they are tired, hurt or bewildered, others through beating themselves up trying to be Superwomen and others because they are crippled with horrifying conviction that anatomy is destiny.

And so it is, but only partly. It is true, women walk differently, bulge differently, throw differently, have a few different organs but not all of the differences are apparent in monthly centrefolds. When I was a teenager a woman could be defined more easily by what she could not do as by what she could. Now centuries of women's self-abnegation are being atoned for. Integrity, delight, commitment, bravery and intelligence are winning through and this new found competence is intoxicating. It embraces taking responsibility for our own health care, appreciating, evaluating and treasuring our bodies in a totally new way.

For too long now we have been dispossessed of the immense knowledge about our bodies, (and thus power) by doctors who are mainly male. Centuries ago the rhizotomists who gathered roots and herbs for medicinal use were generally women. The wild or wise women in early Germany had much in common with the Celtic order of Druidesses. When women lost this control and were condemned to being burned for knowing too much or demoted to the subordinate role of nurse, men began to dominate the medical profession and much of it they designed for their own convenience. Men who have neither vagina or uterus still dominate gynaecology and until recently labour wards were constructed for the convenience of the doctor not the labouring mother.

Indeed a friend was recently told she could do anything she liked in the labour ward provided she didn't get down off the narrow uncomfortable National Health Service bed. I insisted she change hospitals. The freedom to look at the institutions which are created to serve us, critically, intelligently and with strength is vital.

This then is a book about women and their health care needs, written for women, by a woman. It is about the way I perceive women are, not as men or even women would like them to be. The majority of my patients are women and children. It has been my very real delight to work with them over the years, a reciprocation which has been particularly exciting because we have allowed information and feeling to interact. (No one learns very much if they are passive recipients of information.) That the proof of the pudding is in the eating is particularly apposite here. We have learned together about the best way to administer a vaginal douche, about diet, about the myriad different reasons one gets constipated, about simple ways to take care of the skin. Above all we have supported each other by trying to live heroically, rather than traditionally, honouring our innate beauty and power. We have come to understand that ignorance and shame alienate us from ourselves and that such fragmentation stops us from being the whole people we could be.

Wholistic medicine is really the ordinary common sense medicine which has been practised for centuries. It is based on the accurate observation of natural laws. By breaking them we can cause illness and dis-ease. Herbs, like people, differ in their physiological chemistry depending on environmental conditions and this is in spite of the fact that they may be botanically identical. Repeated measurements of the same quantity do not always give identical results because, by its very nature, biological material is variable. To complicate things still further the effect of one particular herb may be altered substantially by the presence of variable amounts of other herbs. Few of the herbal formulae in this book consist of a single herb in isolation and herein lies the fundamental difference between herbal and allopathic medicine. The latter is usually symptomatic in approach, the former looks to treat the patient as a whole not merely a collection of symptoms. But it does so wisely and safely in spite of the fact that allopaths find the variability of herbs confusing, inexact or unpredictable (though practised herbalists who know that herbs like people vary have no such difficulty). Part of the reason for both the efficacy and safety of herbs is the extra ballast which surrounds the concentrated chemical constituents in them. This collection of compounds present in such minute concentration that it is often undetectable by standard techniques not only buffers the action of the whole plant so avoiding the toxic side-effects of its chemical cousins but often promotes the efficient workings of certain enzymes or encourages the development of a good immunological defence system. The tonic herbs like ginseng exercise the subtle effect acting as an adaptogen. Ephedra sinensis (not to be muddled with the American species of ephedra christened 'desert tea') is an alternative example of the buffering constituents in any one herb. It is a natural source of the drug ephedriane used to help asthmatics, but used in this form it also raises the blood pressure. Fortunately, the plant itself, ephedra, contains norephedriane and pseud-ephedrian which has a slightly antagonistic effect to ephedriane so buffering its action. Thus asthma can be helped using a remedy based on the whole plant without us upsetting the patient's blood pressure. The Chinese have used ephedra, which they call Ma Huang, for centuries for precisely this purpose. Digitalis and rauwolfia are among the growing lists of herbs which are now proved to benefit from the balancing action of their many chemical constituents and buffering agents, enabling the body to cope better with the natural plant in its whole state.

Each of us has a unique pattern which fits no one else and *A Woman's Herbal* is designed to cater for differing needs as far as is possible in any book. It begins with preventative medicine advocating diet as the bedrock of all good health and expands with the positive influence radical modification to diet by means of fasting has on health maintenance. It explains how to use herbs for general body maintenance and cleansing, rather like putting yourself in for a five thousand mile service. It describes how to use herbs for emergency treatment as part of a first aid cabinet, how to cultivate and process them and where to buy them if you can't. Just as important it explains which herbs may be contra-indicated and why. It describes simple methods of external care and then goes on to deal with specific female problems ranging from menstrual difficulties to post natal depression, but it does not neglect how to cope with the simplicities of the common cold or athletes foot. It puts the power back where it belongs, into our own hands, so that by learning to understand, accept and be responsible for our bodies and our mental welfare we can really start to fly and appreciate that everything is possible and that never again do we need to settle for anything less than absolutely everything.

I

Diet – the Basis of Health

A good diet is the indispensable bedrock of all preventive and corrective medicine. Those patients who come to see me in the mistaken belief that I am going to behave like an allopathic doctor (i.e. an 'ordinary' western doctor), pat their hand and dispense a herbal remedy instead of a pill to cure all their ills get a jolt when they find out how dependent their treatment is on diet and their willingness to change it. Among their many assets herbs are foods in themselves and serve to supplement and assist the other things that are being ingested.

Dr Roger Williams, the noted biochemist, comes straight to the point.

If in doubt try nutrition first. . . . The most basic weapons in the fight against disease are those most ignored by modern medicine: the numerous nutrients that the cells of our bodies need. . . . Faulty cellular nutrition of one type or another may be the most basic cause of the non-infective diseases – diseases that are at present poorly controlled by medical science.

He is referring here to diabetes, arthritis, the sclerotic diseases, cancers and heart problems. So you appreciate why I make a good diet the cornerstone of any healing programme.

Let's be clear about this. No one diet suits everyone. Our nutritional needs are as different and as individual as our fingerprints. One woman's meat can literally be another's poison.

It is now readily acknowledged that people's nutritional needs will vary according to lifestyle and stage of life, and are affected by such factors as stress, illness, puberty, pregnancy and lactation, the menopause and old age. But what is less clearly understood is that structural and enzymatic differences, which are partially determined by genetics, will determine how you will absorb any nutrients. You may be continually urinating a nutrient away simply because your renal threshold for it is very low, or you may have insufficient intestinal bacteria to ensure the absorption or manufacture of a certain nutrient. Or what Roger Williams calls 'one of the fundamental "wisdoms of the body" . . . the wisdom to eat' may be impaired for any one of myriads of reasons so that you cannot choose food wisely.

My views on diet in general are outlined in detail in *Kitty Campion's Handbook of Herbal Health* and I've subsequently listed the nutritional contents of scores of foods, together with recipes and appropriate advice about their background and selection, in *Kitty Campion's Vegetarian Encyclopaedia* so there is no need to cover this basic ground again here. But there are a few points about food, its selection and preparation which are particularly relevant to women, which I have not covered elsewhere and which do need emphasizing.

Meat

HORMONES IN MEAT
Modern meat rearing now involves administering hormones to animals in the form of ear implants. One of these hormones, zeranol, is a form of oestrogen made from mould called fusarium. This hormone occurs naturally in crops cut in damp weather and, given our miserable climate, the level of this natural hormone in our food can be quite high.

High levels of oestrogen are now known to aggravate cancers of the breast, ovary and lining of the womb. While the level of oestrogen we eat in meat is not that high in itself, if you couple it with the oestrogen already present in women on the pill and pregnant women the balance might just prove damaging.

In addition, a large percentage of women in this country are noticeably zinc-deficient and some animals ingest copper-containing formulae which makes this balance even worse because copper is antagonistic to zinc.

ANTIBIOTICS IN MEAT
Antibiotics have also been used as a growth promoter for forty years and we now get a small but insidious dose of antibiotics in

nearly every meat, dairy product or egg we eat. These kill the benign intestinal bacteria we need for optimum digestion, leaving us wide open to – among other nasties – yeast organisms like *Candida albicans* and consequent infections like thrush.

Dairy Products

MILK

Cow's milk was designed to feed calves. At birth they weigh 70 lb (30 kg) and once their weight has increased tenfold they have reached adolescence and are living off grass alone. This takes less than a year. Humans are designed to increase their weight much more slowly. Many of us do not produce enough lactase to digest cow's milk properly and consequently get wind, indigestion, and mucus and sinus problems.

Pasteurized milk is not the answer. It is vastly deficient in vitamins A, B and C, calcium, iodine and the enzymes that make it more digestible. Homogenized milk isn't the answer either. The tiny globules of fat in it pass through the intestinal wall unaltered and the xanthine oxidase (an enzyme that leads to deterioration of heart function) in these globules is now believed to be one of the major causes of heart failure. Under ordinary circumstances, when the fat globules remain their normal size, xanthine oxidase merely gets excreted harmlessly. In case you are beginning to get hopeful, low-fat milk is not the answer either because the more fat is removed the less calcium is assimilated. By reducing the fat content the fat-soluble vitamins A and D are also proportionately reduced, and these are then often added back synthetically – which is about as silly as putting petrol in a car without wheels, because the fat in milk facilitates the passage of vitamin D into the bloodstream.

Also, butter fat actually protects us against atherosclerosis. The Masai people, whom I used to admire as a child in East Africa, ingest well over half their calories in raw butter fat, and heart disease, cancer and diabetes are rarities among them. Roger Williams in his book *Nutrition Against Disease* details extensive studies providing that non-fat dry milk fed to rats produced atherosclerosis when full-fat did not.

One alternative is raw milk produced by cows certified to be free of disease, but this is difficult to get hold of. An easier alternative is yoghurt or kefir, both of which actually lower cholesterol in the bloodstream. The yoghurt or kefir should ideally be made with sheep's or goat's milk. I bought my own kefir plant back from Istanbul and I feed it daily with one or the other. It is a cousin to yoghurt but has the added advantage of being extremely easy to make and needing no special temperature control. It is a mushroom-like fungus which simply needs to be strained through anything other than metal, washed under cold running water, mixed with any quantity of room-temperature milk and left until the milk turns the consistency of thin yoghurt, which takes about 24 hours – then the whole process is repeated.

Goat's milk contains fat and protein molecules which are much smaller than those in cow's milk, making it easier to digest. Cow's milk takes two hours, goat's only twenty minutes. Sheep's milk, admittedly still a rarity, is better still. For one thing it has no taint and has even smaller fat globules; for another it contains more protein and B vitamins than either of the other two and it freezes beautifully. Greek sheep's milk yoghurt is now widely available commercially.

YOGHURT
All the vegetable gums or gelatins added to commercial yoghurt for thickness actually denature the yoghurt and so invalidate its bacterial content. Be wary of 'no sugar added' yoghurt – it is a labelling which may hide the fact that the fruit added has been previously treated with sugar, and remember that sugar kills acidophilus, the benign flora in yoghurt which helps to protect the intestine. Commercial frozen yoghurt may be ripe with sugar, corn syrup, sodium citrate, polysorbate 80, mono- and di-glycerides, carboxymethyl cellulose – enough artificialities to put a chemical factory to shame! The thickest, creamiest yoghurts often don't have any live yoghurt culture at all. If in doubt read the label and look for the word 'live' or the name of the bacteria in the yoghurt, usually *Lactobacillus bulgaricus* or *Lactobacillus acidophilus*.

CHEESE
Traditional rennet (rennet is used in cheese-making to curdle the milk) comes from calves' stomachs. Vegetable rennet is not

derived from a vegetable source but from chemicals, so when you eat a so-called 'vegetarian' cheese this is what you are eating. Avoid cheeses containing artificial colouring and go for goat's milk and sheep's milk cheeses and those from organic farms. Don't buy Danish feta cheese – it is made from cow's milk with additives in it. Greek feta cheese is exceptionally salty and needs to be soaked overnight in water and then drained. Homemade cottage cheese is best.

Coffee

Coffee drinkers suffer at least twice the incidence of pancreatic cancer suffered by their coffee-shunning sisters and the rate is directly proportional to the amount consumed. This is probably the result of pesticides, most of which dissolve in oil, and coffee is rich in oil. The caffeine in coffee is linked to heart disease, and coffee drinkers suffer from 60 per cent more heart attacks than abstainers if up to five cups a day are drunk, and 120 per cent more when coffee consumption exceeds this level. It causes palpitations, raises blood pressure and cholesterol levels, increases stomach acid secretion, aggravates fibrocystic breast disease and increases the risk of miscarriages, premature births and birth defects. Its psychological effects include insomnia, anxiety, panic attacks, depression and aggravation of schizophrenic psychosis.

The combination of caffeine and sugar in soft drinks like Coca-Cola and Pepsi is particularly insidious because both caffeine and sugar are addictive.

Decaffeinated coffee is not the answer. Trichlorethylene was used to decaffeinate coffee until quite recently when it was proved to be carcinogenic. Now petrol-based solvents are often used instead and I think these are almost certainly going to be proved harmful in the long run too.

The only firm I know which does not use chemicals and which is prepared to divulge exactly how their decaffeinated coffee is processed is Nestlé. Their beans are flushed several times with pressurized hot water which dissolves the caffeine. This then drains away in the liquid. The green beans are then washed and marketed as freeze-dried instant coffee called Descaf. Please remember that even decaffeinated coffee may upset the digestive process because of the amount of tannic acid which remains in it.

The alternatives are grain coffee made from cereals and fruits and readily available in health food shops; chicory coffee; dandelion coffee – not the shop-bought instant stuff which is high in lactose and sickly sweet, but the real root. You can make your own. It requires a little effort but the fresh taste is well worth it.

Dandelion coffee

Harvest the taproots especially carefully on a fine November day when the root is at its richest in inulin. You will need to dig deep and carefully, to avoid gouging them. Shake off any surplus soil, hold them under running water, and while you do so scrub them with a stiff brush until they are clean. Pat dry with a cotton tea towel and split any very thick roots with a stainless steel knife. Lay them on a baking sheet and dry them out in the oven at a low heat. Once a root snaps it is ready. If it merely bends it still has some way to go. I used to use my Rayburn for this but having just moved house I have yet to try drying the roots in my electric oven. I imagine a temperature of about 300°F/150°C/gas mark 2 will be adequate.

You can now store these dried roots until you want to use them. I then roast them in an oven until brown, mill them reasonably finely in a coffee grinder and treat the result in exactly the same way as coffee. Dandelion coffee tastes very bitter, so sweeten it with honey if desired. Always serve it black (I think milk makes it taste decidedly odd). It is wonderful for cleansing and strengthening the liver and so purifying the blood but for medicinal use the freshly scrubbed raw root is much more effective.

Tea

There is twice as much caffeine in tea as in coffee, which makes it a very strong stimulant. The tannin in it curbs hunger pangs and it is so astringent that it inhibits the absorption of iron.

Imported tea contains copper and other impurities. The only alternatives I would recommend apart from herbal teas are green China tea which is actively medicinal and tastes delicious, preferably bought direct from China untreated. I drank it in enormous quantities while in China and found it lowered my body temperature in blistering heat and eased and promoted the digestion of meals (some of which certainly needed the extra help because they contained such exotics as bear's paw, locusts, camel's hoof and moss!).

Bancha tea, which is made from the twig of the tea bush and so contains no caffeine, is superabundant in minerals and available in macrobiotic food shops. Rooibosch tea, which is made from the *Aspalanthus linearis*, has a pleasantly smoky flavour and is rich in vitamin C and trace minerals while being caffeine-free.

Alcohol

The good news is that wine and beer are actually healthy taken in moderation — no more than two drinks daily and these always with meals. Wine is closer in composition to our gastric juices than is any other drink but it may also be loaded with chemicals (none of which need legally be listed on the label). Many asthmatics react severely to the sulphur dioxide used in wine to halt fermentation and kill bacteria. Other common additives include white sugar (manufacturers are permitted up to 53 per cent water and/or sugar in wine). Other additives (a choice of nearly 100 in all) may mean you are virtually drinking a chemical factory, though happily the recent lethal addition of the major constituent of antifreeze was quickly nipped in the bud. To avoid all this I go over to Germany to buy organic wine yearly. It is also available in this country from the supplier listed in the Appendix.

Many beers labour under the same additive problems as wine. Any German beer made according to the 'Bavarian purity decree' is fine and these include Lowenbrau, Lederer-Brau, Spaten, Wuzberger and Hofbrau Bavaria.

Bran

Judging by the enormous quantities of bran many of my patients doggedly chew their way through there is obviously a widespread belief that it is one of the best answers to a constipated maiden's prayer. It is not. The most commonly consumed form of bran is wheat bran and 30 per cent of my patients are wheat-intolerant. Wheat bran scours the delicate lining of the bowel and if a person is constipated it will often make the condition worse not better. High levels of it can inhibit the absorption of iron and other minerals. I far prefer flax-seed ('linseed') or psyllium mixed with plenty of fruit or vegetable juice and taken twice daily between meals, beginning with a teaspoon of seed taken in plenty of liquid and increasing to a tablespoon. These seeds are soft, mucilaginous and don't scour. Linseed has the added advantage of actively deodorizing the bowel with tiny amounts of linamarase, blocking reabsorption. It does not cause bloating or wind even in the very elderly.

To gently correct constipation I will combine the following measures: a bowel cleanse; a high-raw diet where the food is extremely well chewed, grains are avoided completely except in their sprouted form, and plenty of yoghurt or kefir is consumed; colonic massage see Chapter 3); certain yoga positions; regular and vigorous exercise; fasting (see Chapter 2); enemas (see Chapter 6); and 3½ pints (2 litres) water daily in addition to the normal liquid intake.

Artificial Sweeteners

It seems that the phenylalanine component of aspartame used in two top brands of sweetener in the UK, may affect the body's neuro-transmitters.

Dr Pardridge, associate professor of medicine at the University of California, asserts that the US Food and Drugs Agency has seriously underestimated the doses of this sweetener that are likely to be consumed. He asserts that pregnant mothers who unknowingly carry the gene for phenylketonuria are sensitive to phenylalanine and may achieve plasma phenylalanine levels high enough to knock 15 to 20 points from the IQ levels of their children. He also believes that children might become hyperactive and that adult women might experience menstrual changes, and urgently recommends a moratorium on any new products containing aspartame until the dosage and effects can be re-evalued.

His opinion is endorsed by Dr Holtzman, chairman of the Genetics Committee of the American Academy of Paediatrics, who concurs that it seems possible that the highest doses may 'approach the toxic range' for the 10 per cent of the population who carry the phenylketonuria gene. Dr Olney, professor of medicine at Washington University, fears that the effects on children might be quite subtle and develop so insidiously that they are not diagnosed and the cause identified until a generation has been exposed for a number of years. He says:

... because the harm will already have irreversibly occurred before it is recognized and because large numbers of people are potentially at risk, I consider this a serious health problem.

Many soft drink manufacturers use aspartame for their UK diet drinks but the cans do not even carry a warning (as US products are legally obliged to do) that the phenylalanine in as partarme may damage children suffering from phenylketonuria.

A recent study of ninety-five volunteers aged 18–22 in Leeds showed that people actually felt hunger after eating food sweetened with aspartame, an effect which is not very desirable in view of the fact that most people use artificial sweeteners to lose weight or stabilize their weight.

I would suggest that you avoid artificial sweeteners altogether in all forms no matter what their source.

Water

Few people can be unaware that fluoride has been the subject of fierce controversy in the UK in recent years. In every other European country fluoride is banned because it is believed to be a slow-acting poison but in this country local authorities are continuing to fluoridate water, albeit amidst vociferous opposition. Once it is artificially in the water it can only be removed by distillation or ion exchange. Water filters won't do it.

As if this were not worrying enough, the British government has still not acted to satisfy an EEC directive to limit pollutants in drinking water, in spite of the passing of the final deadline in July 1985, and according to the Department of the Environment is not likely to do so in the foreseeable future. There are four pollutants causing particular concern: nitrates from fertilizers; lead; aluminium; and pesticides. Levels of nitrates in water in agricultural areas such as East Anglia and Yorkshire have been rising rapidly and in some areas are well over the limit considered safe by the World Health Organization. High levels have been implicated in infant poisoning and stomach cancer.

Lead is another problem. High levels are clearly linked with brain damage in children, impaired brain function in adults and heart disease, but the government cannot make tap-water levels comply with the EEC directive until it has completed its own programme which won't happen until 1989. This should ensure that local authorities supply water which is unlikely to dissolve lead, but once water reaches the boundaries of your property the responsibility becomes yours and most of the lead gets into water from old-fashioned domestic piping.

The Department of the Environment is still quibbling with the EEC about the exact level of various pesticides to be allowed in water. Apparently aluminium levels will be brought into line — but not yet!

Areas with poor water supplies are primarily in East Anglia, the North and West of England, and Wales and Scotland. Water can also contain chlorine that has not been filtered out once it has done its work, ammonia, sulphates, copper and asbestos, and in one area of the country it recently contained minute shrimp-like creatures. The Oundle Division of Anglian Water naturally made light of the problem, asserting that the treatment needed to flush out these tiny shrimps would 'have no effect on human beings or domestic animals but as fish can be adversely affected, it is advisable that the water in fish tanks or ponds is not changed during the period while the work is being undertaken'. They justified their use of pyrethrin, the substance needed to knock the shrimps out for a while and make them release their otherwise tenacious grip on the side of the pipe (it seems a straight flush would not shift them) with the assertion that this was an organic, naturally occurring biodegradable material.

To purify your water, buy a filtering jug from a health food shop or chemist. An alternative is to drink bottled mineral water. Evian, Volvic, Malvern, Ashbourne and Perrier are all acceptable. Perrier is slightly acidic so it shouldn't be drunk while you are fasting and trying to alkalize your bloodstream.

Lead

Apart from the problem of lead 1 water mentioned above, most tinned food comes in lead-soldered tins so don't buy it. There are a very few companies, such as the manufacturers of the Whole Earth range, which use another, less lethal canning process, and those who do say so on the label round the tin. All food displayed on the pavement next to a busy road will be groaning with lead — don't buy it.

Aluminium

Don't use aluminium kitchen-ware or foil or any of the many products which contain aluminium. These include most table salts, baking powder, antacids, toothpaste, cigarette filters, buffered aspirin, hot-water heaters with aluminium heating elements, and processed cheese. Aluminium is highly toxic. Not only does it create digestive problems but it may be linked with Alzheimer's disease, a form of early senility which can start as young as forty. It has become something of an epidemic in America and now kills more people than cancer, and it is getting that way in Britain too. Use earthenware, glass, china, iron or stainless steel in the kitchen, and greaseproof paper or roasting bags. Aluminium-free baking powder can be made with 1 teaspoon potassium bicarbonate added to 2 teaspoons cream of tartar and 1 teaspoon arrowroot.

Microwaves

It seems that in a few years' time half of all households will own one but I believe that this is another gigantic experiment on the population which will certainly prove to be detrimental in the long run. The Russians have found that chronic exposure to low levels of microwave emission may result in biological changes including a decreased rate of heart muscle contraction, low blood pressure, changes in the blood's composition, thyroid problems, hormone imbalance, alterations to the central nervous system, brain-wave patterns, and behaviour, and a lot of non-specific ailments. There is also a growing suspicion that these ovens lead to a higher rate of breast cancer among those who use them. Currently the regulations governing the safety of microwaves are not stringent enough to protect from leakage.

Gas

This is surprisingly common allergen. If you are prone to allergies like asthma or eczema or get vague headaches it is better to stick to electricity for cooking.

Eating Out

There will undoubtedly be occasions when you simply cannot ignore restaurant food. Having cooked professionally in such places in various parts of the world I have a fairly good idea of what goes on behind the scenes, but it is still possible to work your way through this minefield and enjoy your meal with a clear conscience knowing it is halfway nutritious.

Avoid menus which are overly long and full of complicated, heavily sauced dishes. A short menu with a few simply cooked items is liable to represent good fresh ingredients. Don't eat anything deep fried. Order baked or new potatoes in their skins. Don't patronize places which sell all sorts of different salads with creamy complex dressings. If there are a few salads on the menu, and the greenery looks crisp and undressed and there is nothing canned added, go for these. Ask for the ingredients to make up your own dressings. Otherwise choose the cooked vegetables and specify no butter.

Often I don't bother to read the menu at all. I simply negotiate for what I want. Sometimes the waiters get a little flustered but by being assertive and charming I usually win. I often advise my cancer patients who are on very selective diets to telephone the restaurant in advance and explain the situation and in these instances the chef has always come up trumps. Most imaginative chefs love a challenge! Sometimes I 'phone in advance myself simply offering as an excuse the fact that I am having to follow a special diet for health reasons (which is of course perfectly true). When I go to the theatre or cinema I pack some grapes so that I don't feel deprived in the interval. When I travel by air, as I frequently do, I try and negotiate with the airline in advance but if they come up with something totally inappropriate I have a bag of fruit at the ready and a supply of my three-seed mix (equal parts of pumpkin, sunflower and sesame seeds).

When I visit friends and restaurants I always carry a few herbal tea-bags with me as coffee and tea now literally make me ill.

All of this sounds as if I manage to keep my halo well burnished at all times. Untrue! There are occasions when I leap in feet first and succumb to temptation. Not often but when I do so I make sure I relax, savour every mouthful and really enjoy it, because nothing upsets the digestion more than guilt or worry. And if I am going to succumb I make certain I do this with only one course and one item in that course (usually the dessert course — my Achilles' heel is homemade ice-cream).

Assimilating what you eat

'You are what you eat' would be much more accurately stated as 'You are what you assimilate'. You may be eating the world's most nourishing diet and eliminating with the precision of a sergeant-major but if you are not making full and proper use of that food it is all, literally, a waste of time (and money). I have encountered some people who fill themselves with vitamins and minerals until they are in danger of rattling and who still creep around feeling half dead. This is because there is some organ, gland or system which is damaged, malformed, traumatized or underdeveloped and so unable to function efficiently metabolically. This is further complicated by the fact that your dietary needs are totally different to everyone else's — so your need for vitamin B_{12}, for example, may be several times higher than your neighbour's. There are many things you can do to ensure efficient assimilation.

CHEWING
Proper digestion begins in the mouth. Saliva is permeated with ptyalin which helps to break down starch, so if you gulp your food or talk excessively while eating you won't be able to make full use of it. Chew your food patiently until it is a liquid pulp before swallowing it.

LIQUIDS
These dilute the digestive juices and should not be taken with meals. Drink half an hour before or an hour after a meal. The only exceptions are vegetable and fruit juices which count as a food (and so should be swished round the mouth well to ensure they are mixed with plenty of saliva before swallowing). Herbal teas count as a medicine and may be used to swallow herbal capsules with. Good wine and champagne taken in moderation actually help the digestion by aiding relaxation and so may be taken on high days and holidays with a celebratory meal.

EMOTIONS
The metabolic processes of the body are much more upset by distress, rage, greed, shock, fear, guilt, anxiety, depression, jealousy and grief than by the odd mouthful of naughty food. You need emotional equilibrium to digest your food properly. If you are at all upset miss a meal. If you are upset but feel starving and desperately want to eat sip a small glass of freshly pressed fruit or vegetable juice slowly. Try not to eat to comfort yourself or to relieve tiredness. It's an easy trap to fall into. It stuns me how many people use the family dining-room table as a battleground, and how many children have forkfuls of food forced between their clenched teeth or are constantly admonished to clear their plates. Unhappily, eating everything put in front of you is a destructive habit too many people drag with them into adulthood.

TOO MUCH, TOO OFTEN
Most of us eat too much too often. It takes four hours to empty

the stomach completely, so the ideal eating pattern is a light breakfast at 8 o'clock, a sustaining lunch at 1 o'clock and a light snack at 6 o'clock. (This does not apply if you are hypoglycaemic and need to eat little and often.) If you follow this pattern you won't tax your body's enzymic systems.

PRE-PRANDIAL TITBITS
Don't titivate your jaded appetite with salted snacks or pickles. Salt and vinegar will run down the stomach lining over time. Choose something raw to begin with, such as a piece of fruit or some crudités, which will help to perk up your immune system, avoid digestive leucocytosis (the breakdown of the ability to produce white corpuscles of blood or lymph) and get the gastric juices flowing.

FOOD COMBINING
Proteins are the only food digested in the stomach. The digestion of starchy foods begins in the mouth and ends in the intestines. If you persist in mixing starches and protein together the starches are trapped in the stomach while the protein is digested and the starches ferment and become sour. If you mix acid fruits and starchy foods together it also encourages fermentation and indigestion. There is an excellent book by Doris Grant and Jean Joice which deals with the subject of food combining and is listed in the references at the end of the book.

APPETITE
If you are not hungry don't eat. It sounds obvious but many people eat out of sheer habit.

Digestive tea

    2 parts ginger root
    2 parts fenugreek
    2 parts allspice
    1 part cinnamon
    2 parts dandelion
    1 part plantain
    1 part meadow-sweet
    1 part scullcap

Brew as an infusion (see Chapter 6) and drink 1 cup while eating. This assists the gastric juices, pancreas, liver, stomach and intestines, normalizes stomach acids and helps to remove any excess acid, stops burping and any mucus congestion, soothes the nervous system and tastes spicily palatable.

Supplementation for Optimal Nutrition

I am not a great believer in shop-bought vitamins and mineral supplements because their quality is so suspect. They are generally synthetic and often expensive. It may be true that a molecule of synthetic crystalline ascorbic acid is chemically identical to the ascorbic acid present in rosehips, but the rosehips contain vital accessory factors such as minerals, trace minerals, enzymes and coenzymes as well as minute traces of other probably vital nutrients which we know little about as yet. The substances interact with one another to ensure the full absorption and utilization of the ascorbic acid in a wonderful burst of internal cooperation.

This is true of all herbs. In parsley, for example, the ascorbic acid, vitamin A, essential oils, flavones and various minerals all combine to assist each other to increase the flow of saliva, cleansing the mouth and reducing the bacteria there. Once in the intestine the ascorbic acid and its adjuncts are absorbed very slowly, ensuring that faeces remain soft and so acting as a gentle laxative and an effective diuretic. In an ideal world a balanced diet of fresh, unprocessed foods would supply all our vitamin needs, but unprocessed food is very hard to come by. And it also needs to be remembered that vitamin needs vary with age, stress, illness, pregnancy and alcohol and tobacco intake. The following formulation is a carefully balanced herbal alternative to synthetic vitamin and mineral supplements. It contains the full range of vitamins and mineals, amino-acids and alkaline protein, all of which are easily assimilable.

Herbal mega-multi vitamin and mineral supplement

　2 parts spirulena
　2 parts alfalfa
　2 parts rosehip

2 parts kelp
1 part yellow dock
1 part comfrey
1 part cayenne
1 part Irish moss
1 part Iceland moss
1 part horsetail
1 part parsley
1 part watercress
1 part lobelia

Take two rounded 5 ml teaspoons of the powdered herbs stirred into vegetable juice with each meal. The dose can be adjusted according to need and should therefore be increased for convalescents, pregnant and lactating women, menopausal women and anyone under stress.

Body Talk

You will notice that I haven't given you any hard-and-fast rules about diet. That is because you will find you are wise enough to sort out for yourself what you need to eat and when you need to eat it. It is an extraordinary fact but I have observed it over so many years working with my patients that I know it to be true — once you have cut out all the junk food from your diet and cleared the rubbish from your system your body will tell you what it needs. It is no longer clogged up and weighed down and that powerful and ancient knowing with which all of us are born but which during the growing-up process gets lost under a deluge of rubbishy chemicalized food surfaces again.

Let me give you a case in point. A few months ago I was at a well-known health clinic where I had chosen to fast on fruit for three weeks. On the seventh day I began menstruating and by the eighth day I was feeling so low I actually fainted. Knowing what I do about fasting, I appreciated that the eighth-day was 'a crisis of acidosis' but I was losing blood at a very fast rate (which is unusual for me) and I can never remember fainting in my life. When I came to, I had a desperate craving for red grape juice. I told the nurse about it who adamantly refused to let me add it to my fruit diet because, as she put it, 'All diets have been very carefully thought out and are totally adequate.' She was wrong. No one diet will ever suit everyone under all circumstances. Red grape juice is high in fructose and iron and that is exactly what I needed that day because my body wisely told me so.

I have known some people vomit up even a cup of herbal tea at the beginning of diet reform. This is not instinctive body talk. It is because the body is so toxic and the digestion so battered that it cannot deal even with the simplest bit of pure nutrition and in this instance I get the patient to start with just a few teaspoons of the tea and graduate from there. I must emphasize that accurate body talk only begins once you have cleaned the body up. At first your inner voice will come in whispers and fits and starts because a new way of eating is rather like learning to ride a bike. You wobble about a lot and fall off several times but when you doggedly remount and keep wheeling you eventually get the hang of it and finally the speed, once you know how, is wonderfully exhilarating! At that point you won't have to rely on any books or gurus – you will find out exactly what you always wanted to know about what suits *you*.

The Tortoise and the Hare

I will offer you a final piece of advice on diet reform I always give my patients. *Don't do it all at once* unless you have phenomenal will power. Alter one aspect of your diet at a time. Choose to give up, say, coffee to start with and expect to feel exhausted initially as you come off all those adrenal stimulants. There is plenty of herbal help near to cleanse and support the body while you do so.

You will notice something very intriguing when you transfer your allegiance to an imaginative, balanced, wholefood, predominantly raw diet. Your taste-buds will get sharper and fussier and you will actually feel nauseated not just naughty when you eat foods which don't suit you. Or you will get headaches, aches and pains, a rash, diarrhoea, bloodshot eyes or halitosis and you will decide that it is just not worth paddling in your own poison.

Don't, as you change your eating habits, let the smell of burning martyr's flesh pervade your house. Try not to become a fanatic but on the other hand don't let other people's opinions bother or sway you. It's amazing, but I suppose it's human nature, just how unhelpful friends can be when they see you changing. A lot of mine begged me to stay my sweet, round, cuddly self when I lost a lot of weight. I think the change disconcerted them and made them feel that my character would change with it. For better or for worse it hasn't!

One of the quickest and most satisfying ways to embark on a new way of eating and cleanse your system quickly is to fast. Read on . . .

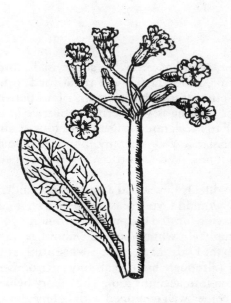

2

The Joy of Fasting

Why Fast?

Otto Buchinger, who has probably supervised more fasts than any other doctor, called fasting the royal road to healing, and judging by the effect fasting has on many of my patients I have to agree with him. Fasting is wonderfully effective in emergencies and works well to accelerate the healing of long-term illnesses. It can help to rebalance you mentally, physically, spiritually and emotionally. Sounds like a tall order? Not when you consider the logic of it.

If your car suddenly developed a nasty rattle under the bonnet at high speed wouldn't you sensibly pull over and check the engine? And having located the problem wouldn't you switch the engine off completely while you went about repairing it? The same applies to the body. Many illnesses are firmly rooted in poor dietary habits (although biological and environmental factors have to be taken into account too). The theory behind fasting is that the body comes well equipped with competent mechanisms for incinerating and eliminating nutritional waste as well as the toxic effects of stress, grief and anger, which often have more to do with the bedrock of illness than does any other factor. The digestive process uses up 30 per cent of the total body energy, so if the digestive system is placed in a complete state of rest, it can concentrate entirely on detoxification and healing.

Fasting is also invaluable preventive medicine. Not only does it help the body to maintain peak fitness by periodically unburdening itself of accumulated waste, but it nips minor health problems in the bud, decelerates the ageing process, if done regularly stabilizes body weight, and helps to prepare the body to utilize nutrition far more effectively after the fast is broken.

The Mechanics of Fasting

At any one time a quarter of our body's cells are in the process of growth, half are at the zenith of their working powers, and the remaining quarter are dying and being replaced. Only by speedy and efficient elimination of these dead cells can the building and growth of fresh cells be stimulated. Fasting actually accelerates the elimination of dead cells and speeds up the building of new healthy cells. This may sound decidedly peculiar in view of the fact that so little nourishment (or in a water fast none at all) is ingested but it is a proven physiological fact. Protein levels in the blood remain constant and normal because the proteins are being constantly decomposed and resynthesized for alternative use. The amino-acids (the building blocks of protein) in the old dead cells, far from being wasted, are released and reused in the process of building new cells.

The cleansing capacity of all the eliminative organs of the body is vastly increased. For instance the concentration of discarded toxins in the urine can be increased up to ten times, and an over-burdened liver can dump its waste six times more quickly than usual, especially when assisted by a certain enemas and poultices (of which more later).

Fasting and Fat

Fasting is really remarkably easy. I find it easier than dieting because it requires less menu preparation and eliminates the possibility of choice, and hence temptation! However it is not the quickest way to lose weight. Fasting for more than a day actually lowers the metabolic rate and the spectacular amount of weight that is lost during the initial days of a fast are merely the result of the liver dumping glycogen and the adjustment of water levels in the body. A substantial percentage of the weight loss during a long fast is rapidly regained once normal eating is resumed – reassuring news to my very thin patients who fear they are going to vanish down the plughole but not good for the fat ones.

If you want to lose weight, a diet consisting of 70 per cent raw food and careful food combinations is ideal, coupled with regular exercise. But fasting is a wonderful way to introduce yourself to such a diet, partly because it shores up will power and shrinks the stomach so that smaller helpings will do, and partly because the digestion and utilization of any subsequent food are greatly enhanced and glandular chemistry and hormonal secretions are stimulated.

Last year I went on a three-week grape fast and lost 12 lb (5 kg) but, having quickly regained nearly half of that when I embarked on new and better eating habits, I then went on to lose a further 2 stone (12 kg) and the weight loss has remained permanent. This year I went on a three-week fruit fast, choosing a different fruit each day, and lost 7 lb (3 kg). A couple of pounds have since been regained but the rest of the loss has been permanent.

How to Fast

Don't fast on water alone, particularly if you have never fasted before. It is a miserable experience for bodies groaning with toxins and the particularly potent ones, the result of ingesting insecticides and poisonous metals, pour into the system so rapidly that you will finish up drowning in your own poison. It is much better to choose either one type of fruit (a mixture will decrease the potency of the fruits' digestive enzymes) or alkaline juices.

FRUIT FASTING

Purists will insist that eating fruit is not strictly fasting and it is true that the digestive organs are not allowed to rest as much as if only liquids were being processed. But eating fruit certainly ensures the discriminate incineration of old tissues (leaving tissues that are ageing but still useful) which is the strict requirement of fasting. Besides which, fruit fasting is good for first-timers who are nervous about going the whole way, and especially beneficial for anyone suffering from chronic constipation. In this case the colon actually needs something rich in fibre to bite on to encourage peristalsis (the automatic wave-like movements by which food is propelled along it), and fruit passes rapidly through the system, requiring very little action by digestive enzymes to make use of it. Most people make the mistake of not eating enough fruit on a fruit fast and then wonder why they get hungry or irritable. The secret of successful fasting is to eat as much of your chosen fruit as you can without being ridiculous about it. As the fast lengthens appetite diminishes, but ensure that, even on a long fast, you eat six servings of fruit daily. Aim for somewhere between 4 and 6 pounds of fruit a day depending on your body weight (less if you are tiny, more if you are not). Chew each piece of fruit slowly and thoroughly until every last drop of juice is extracted before swallowing it, and eat all the fruit including the skin and the seeds unless the skin is obviously inedible (as with bananas or pine-apple). The only bits you are allowed to discard are inedible pips like cherry stones and woody stalks (on apples and grapes, for example). If you can't manage your 4–6 lb (2–3 kg) of fruit daily, juice the remainder and sip it slowly before bed.

Eat several portions of your chosen fruit every 2 hours and let your digestion rest in-between. Do not drink anything whatso-ever with your fruit, not even water. This will dilute the digestive enzymes and so make the fruit a less potent healing tool. You may drink as much mineral water between the fruit as desired but never closer to the fruit than half an hour. If there is a history of deeply entrenched constipation drink a mug of hot purified water on rising and retiring with a slice of well-scrubbed lemon in it to make it more palatable.

VEGETABLE FASTING

I don't prescribe vegetable fasting often simply because most people find it very difficult to chew vast quantities of their chosen raw vegetable (although chomping away at lots of raw carrots is an excellent way to massage the gums back to good health). Also, as no seasoning in any form, except a squeeze of fresh lemon juice, is allowed with your vegetables, some taste-buds rebel at the monotony of undressed raw celery or cauliflower. The only vegetables which may be cooked are beetroot (good for anaemia), asparagus (for flushing out the kidneys), pumpkin and its seeds (for deworming), and artichokes (to cleanse the liver). Beetroot is better well scrubbed and baked rather than boiled (eat the skin too if it is chewable). Drink the water in which the asparagus was cooked too.

All fruits and vegetables must be meticulously washed, if necessary in hot water, before ingestion, and should be absolutely ripe, having reached the perfect state of their 'balsamic moment' as the sixteenth-century herbalists used to put it. Try to use organically grown produce (for suppliers see the contact address in the Appendix.) The same rules which apply to fruit fasting apply to vegetable fasting. Never mix fruits and vegetables. Fruits are much more vigorous and abrasive cleansers than vegetables and they don't marry well together.

JUICE FASTING

Having tried and enjoyed a few fruit and vegetable fasts you can now graduate to juice fasting. Juices are particularly beneficial because you can ingest so much more in terms of quantity and therefore absorb more vitamins, trace elements, minerals and enzymes. Fruit juices maintain a stable electrolyte balance, ensuring that the circulation remains stable. Water taken alone has the dangerous capacity to distort the circulation. Juices are easily assimilated and do not put a strain on the digestion. They do not stimulate the secretion of hydrochloric acid in the stomach (particularly important for those with ulcers or tender stomach linings). They contain an unidentified factor which stimulates microelectric tension in the body and is responsible for the cells' capacity to absorb the nutrients from the bloodstream and so promotes the effective excretion of metabolic waste. One expert on fasting, Dr Berg, is convinced that juices actually *increase* the healing effect of fasting and believes that the concentrated sugars in juices strengthen the heart.

Try to drink 1 fl oz (30 ml) juice for every pound (roughly, 0.5 kg) of your body weight every day. If this is impossible dilute the juice in proportions of half and half with mineral water. Yes, you have done your calculations correctly! You may well be drinking a gallon (4.5 litres) of liquid a day and this is as it should be. The more liquid you take in, the quicker you flush out all the accumulated toxins and the less possibility there is of retaining water, because mineral water and juices act as natural diuretics.

If possible juices should be raw and freshly pressed from well-washed fruit. The most effective juicing machines are those that spin juices out centrifugally and operate continuously. If you haven't got a juicer, buying organic bottled juices is an alternative, but an expensive one. Juices from citrus fruits can be hand-pressed, though this is rather hard work. Juices should be served at room temperature and pressed as needed (to minimize oxidation) and they should be 'chewed' before swallowing. You don't actually have to move your teeth to do this, just swish them well around the mouth to ensure that they are mixed with plenty of saliva before swallowing.

What to Fast On

You don't have to stick to the same juice or fruit for several days running, and indeed it may be unwise to do so simply because of boredom. Much as I love grapes I couldn't look another grape in the eye for six months after my prolonged grape fast last year! But based on the Hippocratic principle of food being your medicine, remember that juices and their fruits will actively heal certain conditions in the body. My first rule is to choose a fruit from your own area. By and large apples will suit those who live in temperate climates, but because I could get hold of local organically grown grapes I chose these, not least because they are the nearest fruit in nature to our own blood chemistry and so make a superb blood purifier. They are also laxative (I used to have the world's most cositive bowel) and they are excellent for catarrhal conditions.

JUICES RECOMMENDED FOR HEALING SPECIFIC AILMENTS

Anaemia
Two teaspoons each of spinach juice and parsley juice, added to a glass of carrot juice or black grape juice (or an equivalent amount of black grapes); or beetroot juice with 1 teaspoon each of garlic juice and hawthorn berry juice added per glass.

Asthma
Equal parts of comfrey juice, horseradish juice and garlic juice, making up 1 teaspoon in all, added to a glass of carrot juice or beetroot juice.

Cellulite
A glass made up of 2 parts celery juice and 1 part beetroot juice with 1 teaspoon watercress juice added; or a glass of water-melon or asparagus juice.

Chronic catarrh
Grape juice (both black and white grapes will do); or equal parts of carrot juice and turnip juice.

Constipation
One teaspoon of each of the following juices: garlic, onion, watercress, dandelion, added to 1 glass made up of equal parts carrot juice, beetroot juice, celery juice and cucumber juice.

Depression
Juice made from well-ripened bananas; or pomegranate juice; or mangoes or their juice.

Diarrhoea
Stewed blueberries or their juice.

Eczema
Blackcurrants; or black grapes or their juice.

Emphysema
Equal parts of carrot juice, parsnip juice, watercress juice and potato juice; or equal parts of orange juice and lemon juice diluted half and half with a strong decoction (see Chapter 6) of rosehip tea.

Gout and arthritis
Black-cherry juice; or equal parts of carrot juice, beetroot juice, celery juice and potato juice with 1 teaspoon parsley juice and 2 teaspoons of the juice from sprouted alfalfa added per glass.

High blood pressure
Any citrus juice or a combination of them; or equal parts of carrot juice and spinach juice with 1 teaspoon each of comfrey juice, parsley juice, onion juice and/or garlic juice added per glass.

Hypoglycaemia
Equal parts of string-bean juice, celery juice and cucumber juice with 1 teaspoon each of garlic juice, watercress juice and juice from sprouted fenugreek added per glass.

Kidney disorders

Equal parts of carrot juice and celery juice with 1 teaspoon each of birch-leaf juice and watercress juice added per glass. If birch leaf is unobtainable add ½ teaspoon horseradish juice instead. For water retention eat water-melon and its seeds.

Leg ulcers

Carrot juice with ½ teaspoon garlic juice and 1 teaspoon comfrey juice added per glass.

Low blood pressure

Pineapples or grapes or their juice; or celery and potato juice in equal parts with 1 teaspoon radish juice added per glass.

Obesity

Pineapple juice (or pawpaw juice) with ½ teaspoon powdered spirulena added per glass. Do not add the latter if you are prone to high blood pressure or chronic lymph congestion.

Stomach disorders

Equal parts of carrot juice, tomato juice, celery juice and potato juice. Gall-bladder inflammation: eat plenty of boiled artichokes (the soft tip and the hearts only) or drink equal parts of carrot juice and beetroot juice, adding 1 teaspoon dandelion-leaf juice and 1 teaspoon radish juice per glass.

Insomnia

Equal parts of carrot juice, celery juice and lettuce juice; or mango juice.

Supplementation and Drugs during Fasting

If you have been on allopathic medicine for some time you should not stop taking it while fasting. You may have to reduce it to only a third or a quarter of the normal dose because it will take effect much more efficiently in the system, but stopping it altogether would be very foolhardy.

Some 'authorities' suggest vitamin, mineral and other supplementation in a fast but I am adamantly against this because it merely forces the body's pace and overexcites the system. Fasting is a natural process and should be done at a normal rhythm. One of the benefits of fasting is that it forces you to acknowledge the true rhythms of your body not the ones you inflict on it with artificial stimulants. The only addition I'll allow my fasting patients is a cup of herbal tea (made with a tea-bag or a sprinkling of herbs, *not* brewed to medicinal strength), sweetened with a little honeycomb. Contrary to popular myth, blood sugar does not drop markedly during fasting but body temperature does, and something hot taken internally will help to raise it. So, of course, will plenty of warm clothes and sensible exercise.

Side-effects of Fasting

Prolonged fasts follow a typical pattern. The body will use all the eliminative channels, minor and major, to excrete waste, and this process will manifest itself right from the first day in bad breath, headaches and a furry tongue. Other side-effects include changes in body odour, dandruff, spots, more ear wax than usual, coughing up lots of phlegm, and heavier vaginal secretions (or if you are having a period it may be an exceptionally heavy one). Don't be ladylike. Spit out the phlegm into a handkerchief, don't swallow it. Use water treatments (see Chapter 6), skin brushing (see Chapter 3) and air baths to encourage elimination through the skin. Do not use an antiseptic mouthwash; instead, scrub your tongue with a toothbrush often, and chew a clove, a piece of raw liquorice root or some citrus pips. Don't block your pores with deodorants, oils, lotions or masks. Use cotton-wool buds to clean the ears. Increased liquid intake will minimize headaches, as will drops of lavender oil massaged into each temple.

You may not experience any of these side-effects, in which case don't get despondent and think that the fast is not working for you. It is. It simply means that you have less toxic waste to get rid of than most and that your body is offloading it more comfortably through another channel you may not readily notice such as the kidneys.

During the first two or three days of a fast you will be hungry because the food-conditioned reflex leucocytosis is generally increased, but after the third day this will drop off sharply as acidosis (an acid condition of the blood) increases, and during days four and five and eight or nine the taint of acetone on the breath can be quite noticeable. Acetone is also excreted in the urine but the alkalinity of plenty of fruit and vegetable juices will soften this effect. Generally on the thirteenth day there is an acetonic crisis when the ketones in the blood serum soar to exceptionally high levels and you may not feel at all well. I normally advise a fair amount of exercise, plenty of rest and particular attention to the external aids such as skin brushing and enemas suggested later in the chapter, but this is especially important on day thirteen.

After this the tongue generally loses its furriness and the skin and breath start to smell less acidic, and the time to stop fasting is when the appetite reappears spontaneously. The biochemical dynamics of fasting follow the same pattern whether you are mentally or physically ill or healthy.

Fasting and Sex

Generally the longer the fast the less sexually active you will feel, but on short fasts I have observed that women tend to feel more enthusiastic about love-making and get more satisfaction from it. Once a long fast is broken, many women have been greatly surprised that sexual appetite comes back with renewed vigour. Certainly I have noticed that after a series of prolonged fasts menstruation becomes regular and metabolic and ovarian problems are greatly improved.

How Long Should You Fast?

If you have never fasted before, begin by choosing just one day a week to fast on and keep to the same day every week if you can. The body feels comfortable with a natural rhythm and the herbs you will be taking when you are not fasting are, in my experience, utilized most efficiently by the body in a seven-day rhythmic cycle in which you take them for six days weekly and rest on the seventh day.

Once you are feeling more adventurous you might like to embark on a three- or four-day fast which will give your body the chance to do some really effective deep cleansing. Don't attempt anything longer than this without supervision from a qualified person well experienced with fasting. I am not in favour of two-day fasts. I liken them to the uncomfortable and unsatisfactory feeling of building up to an orgasm but never actually climaxing. They are a twilight zone between the dumping of glycogen from the liver which happens within twelve hours and the build-up to acidosis but never quite reaching it which leaves the body teetering uncomfortably.

I usually fast for three or four consecutive days monthly, and in the spring greatly look forward to a three-week fast, but would advise a maximum of only two long fasts a year. The longest fast I have ever supervised was for an epileptic patient, a forty-two-day one on carrot juice, and one of the welcome side-effects was a complete healing of deep, weeping leg ulcers which had been present for twenty years.

Aids to Fasting

Always get yourself into a stable and positive mental state before fasting. If you embark on any fast, no matter how short or long, full of fear and misery or feeling like a masochist, you will undoubtedly fail. The only unsuccessful fast I have ever done was one which lasted for six days and was undertaken without adequate preparation and in a fit of depression and exceptional busyness. Never again! True, I have cajoled mentally ill patients into fasting where by dint of using my will power not theirs they have succeeded, but this is exceptional and does not fall within the scope of this book. (Certainly I have found fasting very helpful for treating phobias, neurotic anxiety and depression.)

Skin-brush (see Chapter 3) regularly morning and evening. Wear only natural fabrics at all times and sleep in natural-fabric bedding. Walk barefoot on grass, sand or soil for five or ten minutes very day. It helps the circulation of the whole body and grounds its static electricity, so calming and refreshing it. Walking on grass which is covered with the morning dew is particularly beneficial for people whose nervous system needs regenerating. There is an ancient Greek legend which recounts the story of the giant Antaeus who, as the son of Gaea (the strength-giving Mother Earth) derived his strength from her. It seems his enemy could only beat him at wrestling when he realized that, whenever Antaeus touched the ground, he recovered his strength, but whenever he could be raised off the ground it deserted him. The ancient Greeks obviously knew much more about the rejuvenating effects of barefoot walking than we do. Air-bath for a few minutes daily, exposing the whole body naked to the air while lying in the shade. Fresh air accelerates wound healing and encourages the skin to breathe properly. Take time to breathe properly and deeply.

Follow the natural rhythm of the day, getting up when the sun rises and taking a rest shortly after it sets. Most people need more sleep anyway during a fast, at least in the initial stages. If you only have one opportunity to rest during the day, do so before midday when the liver is still very active. The liver bears the brunt of cleansing during a fast and is at its most active between midnight and midday. Apply a herbal poultice (see Chapter 6) to the liver and lie down. The former will increase blood flow to the liver by 20 per cent, the latter by a further 40 per cent, so greatly easing its burden.

Take an enema (see Chapter 6) before bed, and if you can on rising as well, every day of your fast. This is by far the quickest and most efficient way to cleanse the colon. If you are just fasting on juices don't get complacent and think that the colon will have nothing to excrete. One of its functions is to act in much the same way as the skin does, drawing excretions from the body through the intestinal wall. My forty-two-day fast patient was still having two or three regular bowel movements daily and producing all sorts of interesting waste in his enema water.

Don't watch television, and be selective about the things you read. Fasting is also a form of spiritual cleansing and if you fill yourself with mental rubbish it will leach your emotional energy and may even give you bad dreams. One of the great benefits of fasting is that everything becomes heightened as your body cleanses itself: the taste-buds pick up every nuance of flavour; your sense of smell becomes wonderfully refined; colours get brighter; sounds more distinct; touch more sensitive. Don't cloud this increasing awareness, whether it be with the media, cigarettes or supplements.

Exercise daily, preferably by taking long brisk walks, well wrapped, unburdened and breathing deeply. The lymphatic system will slow down rapidly as the metabolic rate drops and skin-brushing and walking will speed it up and so help it to gather up its waste and dump it efficiently.

Use extra aids like poultices, fomentations, massage, water treatment and reflexology appropriate to the condition being treated.

Breaking Fast

George Bernard Shaw said, 'Any fool can go on a fast but it takes a wise man to break it properly.' No matter how brief or prolonged your fast, make it a golden rule never to overburden the digestive system when you break it. Break your fast by slowly chewing a single ripe apple, or, if your teeth aren't up to it, grate the apple first; eat all of it, core and pips included. For lunch, eat a bowl of mixed fruit salad or lightly steamed vegetables but not both, and drink a few glasses of fruit or vegetable juices during the course of the morning. In the evening eat soupy grains like lentils, millet or buckwheat, liberally seasoned with herbs. Spend as long breaking your fast as you did doing it. If, for example, you have just completed a four-day fast you might introduce dairy products on the second day after breaking it, heavier wheat products on the third, and chicken and fish on the fourth.

Unsuitable Candidates for Fasting

The very elderly, fragile or emaciated.
Those with weak hearts.
Psychotics.
Pregnant women.
Those with TB.
Those suffering from exopthalmic goitre.
People with physically active careers like gymnasts.
Diabetics.

Hypoglycaemics may fast but are best on grapes and need 500 mg of vitamin B_6 and one strong B-complex tablet daily while doing so. The glucose tolerance curve of a hypoglycaemic will certainly be normal at the end of a twenty-one-day fast. Those who are dubious about fasting will undoubtedly meet failure simply because of their negative attitudes.

In an emergency some of the people listed above may fast but they must be guided by a qualified person well versed in supervising fasts.

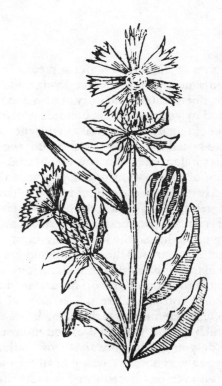

3

Cleansing Vital Organs

Elimination

Most of what goes in should come out somewhere. You can be eating the world's most wonderful diet, living a life of quiet ease and naturalness, but if your eliminatory organs don't disgorge the debris left behind by your metabolic building processes you're in trouble. Regular elimination is as vital as efficient assimilation.

So if you have fasted for a while to clean out the debris, what then? For perfect balanced health you will need to consider the various avenues of elimination and make sure that they are working properly for you on a long-term regular basis. And please go at it gently. Don't start cleansing all six channels at once. (In case you are wondering, the six channels are the lymphatic system, the lungs, the liver, the skin, the kidneys and the bowel.) I am not a great believer in the old-fashioned purge favoured by so many herbalists; for one thing it may leave you so weak and depleted that it puts you off natural medicine for ever. For another, what you assimilate is just as vital as what you eliminate. You can determine which channels are working well for you and which are not with a bit of common sense. Are you constipated or do you get diarrhoea? Do you suffer from water retention? Do you sweat horribly, or not at all even with vigorous exercise? Do you ever feel liverish or get indigestion? Do you suffer from swollen glands, earaches, sore throats, colds? Do you get spots, dandruff, bad breath?

If you want your needs fine-tuned arrange a consultation with a well-trained iridologist (see the contact address in the Appendix). Such a person, by examining your eyes under magnification together with lots of close questioning, will be able to determine your inherited and acquired tendencies towards health and disease, your general bodily condition and the state of every organ in your body. Certainly iridology is the only science I know of that can reliably tell you the state of your lymphatic system and, what is more, warn you of problems there ten or fifteen years ahead; and considering that the breakdown of the lymph system is at the forefront of so many of the serious illnesses occurring in the last decades of life, it is as well to nurture it and keep it in good shape.

The Lymphatic System

This can best be described as the body's vacuuming system. Unlike the blood circulation, it doesn't have the heart to act as the pump; it moves lymphatic fluids around the body through the action of muscles and the lungs, through a one-way valve system, collecting poisons as it goes and disposing of them through the bladder, bowels, lungs and skin. The lymphatic vessels are particularly concentrated in the groin, behind the knees, in the armpits and under the chin, but they spread like a gossamer network of tubes about the diameter of a needle throughout the body, covering every area except the central nervous system. Lymph vessels house a vast population of white blood cells all bent on attacking and ingesting invaders and cleaning out waste. Different types have different specialized roles. The B lymphocytes produce antibodies which immobilize the invader when it comes, whether it be from chemical or bacterial sources. The T-cells actively hunt for foreign invading cells, bacteria, fungi, viruses and allergens by producing lymphokins and macrophages. Between them they act as a good policing team ensuring that your auto-immune system is doing what it should. If they falter, lymphatic statis occurs, and one of the lymphatic nodules swells up with poisonous waste or metallic residue. What you feel is a lump, and you may see a bleeding or enlarged mole. By the time you spot this it means your auto-immune system is on its belly, not just its knees and needs very urgent attention.

The lymphatic system can grind almost to a complete halt if you are constantly exposed to heavy metal and industrial chemicals – breathing them in, putting them on your skin or eating them. It may sound like a frightening scenario but there are plenty of simple ways in which you can assist your lymphatic system.

EXERCISE

Vigorous exercise acts as a powerful pump for the lymph glands and the body heat you generate burns up any excessive fat being marshalled in the lymph vessels. The best way to get the lymph moving is to trampoline on one of those mini trampolines 3 or 4 feet across, but please don't use one of these if you are prone to prolapse. I am seeing an alarming number of women in my clinic who have taken up trampoline rebounding with a vengeance and are aggravating prolapse bladders, wombs and colons. Given this warning, the up-and-down movement of trampolining, together with the unique acceleration–deceleration effect, changes the force of gravity in your body as no other exercise can, putting the lymphatic and blood circulation systems under intense rhythmic pressure. This stimulates the dumping of wastes from all the cells into the intestinal fluid which the lymph system obligingly picks up and flushes away. There is an added bonus – the oxygen you breathe in encourages the on going purification of your whole system.

Your muscles have got to be in fairly good shape before you start any kind of rigorous exercise, so if in doubt begin with long brisk walks, really striding out and swinging your arms. You can graduate to running if you are very strong, providing you keep to soft surfaces like grass – cement or tarmac can be very shocking to your internal organs. Swimming long steady laps solves this problem altogether as you are comparatively weightless in water.

SKIN BRUSHING

This is a wonderfully effective way of moving the lymph from the superficial vessels round the body as well as softening and freeing up any hardened, impacted lymph mucus from the nodes. Five minutes of skin brushing is the equivalent of twenty-five minutes of jogging, not of course as far as the heart is concerned, but as far as the lymphatic system goes. It is not a lazy-girl substitute for exercise and must be done as well as, not instead of. You may notice when you begin your skin brushing that lots of Vaseline-like jelly appears in your faeces initially. This is lymph mucus.

For complete instructions on skin brushing see page 49. When you are skin brushing in order to ginger up the lymphatic system, move always towards the lymph nodes in long, strong, sweeping strokes. So the legs will be brushed upwards towards the groin, paying special attention to the top of the feet and back of the knees; arms will be brushed upwards to the armpits, sweeping down to the heart over the top of the breasts; the neck will be brushed from behind the ears, crossing over the top of each breast to the main lymph ducts in the armpits in one long stroke.

FACIAL MASSAGE

As it is inadvisable to brush the face to stimulate the lymphatic system, I'd suggest you do this with your fingers, which is just as effective. Start with your forehead; with the whole length of the fingers resting on the skin pull outwards from the centre, using both hands in one long stroke down to the cheek-bones. If the skin turns slightly red so much the better. Then pinch the eyebrows firmly between thumb and forefinger, beginning half an inch from the beginning of the eyebrow and going out to the top of the cheek-bone to meet the hairline. Then, using your thumbs only, begin right in the inner corner of the eye by the nose. Go outwards to the cheek-bone, pressing into the skin hard, lifting, then pressing again. Work outwards to the top of the ear. Repeat, following the same line but slightly lower down the face, and follow the same pattern until you reach the area over the mouth. At this point use the index finger and thumb. Press and lift towards the ears with the index finger over the top of the lips and the thumb beneath the bottom lip. Now repeat it but lower down, just above and below the chin along the jaw line, working out to the bottom of the ear. Repeat each pattern across the face at least five times and follow the facial lymph massage with the neck-to-armpit cross-brushing.

LYMPH-CLEANSING HERBS

Allow yourself several months to break down impacted lymph mucus. Herbs which are particularly effective are those high in iron with good traces of copper. Echinacea, nettle, golden-seal, poke root, cleavers, marigold, red clover, plantain, myrrh and bayberry bark are all suitable, and as a tremendous amount of rubbish gets thrown out into the bloodstream during a lymph cleanse, it is as well that many of these also act as fine blood

Facial Lymph Massage

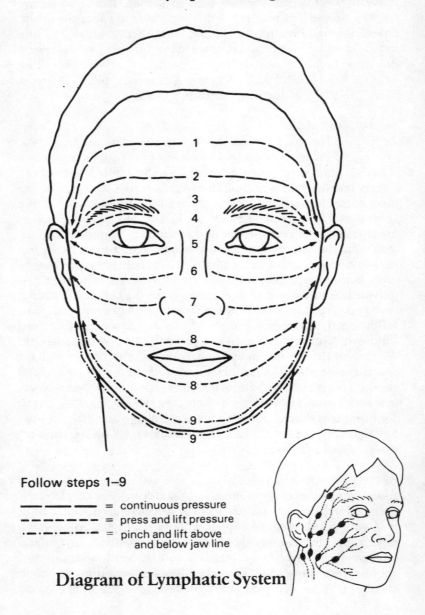

1

2

3

4

5

6

7

8

8

9

9

Follow steps 1–9

— — — — = continuous pressure

- - - - - = press and lift pressure

-·-·-·- = pinch and lift above
and below jaw line

Diagram of Lymphatic System

cleansers. Echinacea actively helps the production of white blood cells and is the supreme lymph cleanser.

Deep lymph formula

2 parts echinacea
2 parts mimosa gum
1 part red clover
1 part nettles
1 part poke root
1 part blue flag
1 part plantain
1 part cayenne

Take three size 'O' capsules of the finely powdered herbs three times daily before meals.

A DIET FOR THE LYMPH SYSTEM
Don't clog your lymph system with red meat, dairy products, sugar, anything artificial, alcohol or fried food. A diet which is superabundant in fresh fruits, dark-green leafy vegetables, sprouted seeds, nuts and a few grains and pulses is ideal.

The Lungs

Count the number of times you breathe in and out for the next minute. If you are sitting quietly it should be somewhere between ten and fifteen times. If you got up and ran around the block you'd double or treble that rate. Your lungs are constantly on the move, flushing out carbon dioxide and carbonic acid wastes, which coalesce in the tissues throughout the body after the nervous system has jettisoned them. Efficient lungs will greatly ease the load of the other eliminative channels and encourage waste elimination. Conversely, sloppy breathing will result in low vitality, and acceleration of metabolic disorders and degeneration of the tissues all over the body. Most pathological changes in these tissues can be prevented if they are constantly surrounded by oxygen. We are, in the deepest and truest sense, what we breathe, and proper breathing is the best preventative medicine of all.

The problem is that most of us forget how to breathe once we get out of nappies. Watch a toddler breathing and you will see her belly rising and falling. None of that stomach in, chest out, shoulders back business for her! Learn to breathe deep not high. Women are particularly prone to moving their shoulders up and down rather than drawing breath into the lungs so deeply that the chest ribs are lifted up and out and the stomach muscles well outwards.

HOW TO BREATHE PROPERLY

Start by improving your posture. Stand and sit tall and when you lie down ensure you are well stretched out. Keep your head well up and don't tuck your chin in or let it stick out. You can check your posture by standing barefoot against a wall without a skirting board. Now try and flatten the whole length of your spine against the wall, keeping the back of your head against it too. Stretch up and breathe out deeply. Take a step away from the wall holding this position – this is how you should stand and walk.

If you suffer from breathing problems, brisk, sustained walking punctuated with plenty of short rests is the best type of exercise. You can consciously work to improve your lung capacity: breathe in while you walk four paces, hold your breath for a further four steps (if it feels uncomfortable let it go – don't explode!), then breathe out slowly with control for six paces. As you improve, gradually increase the count. Swimming gently and consistently is also good but do remember to shower carefully afterwards as chlorine is intensely poisonous.

SMOKING ACTIVE AND PASSIVE

I know I don't have to remake the wheel and tell you what smoking does to you, but perhaps I should observe that the message doesn't seem to be getting through to women. While the proportion of men smoking fell by 27 per cent between 1977 and 1982, the proportion of women smoking over the same period fell by only 20 per cent and those who persisted consumed an average of 13 per cent more cigarettes. The mortality rate for lung cancer in women is escalating and by the end of this century is expected to overtake breast cancer as the major cause of cancer deaths in women.

If you feel you'd rather die than give up smoking there is a middle way to wean you off it. Try herbal smoking mixtures. Honeyrose make one (available in health food shops). I am not implying that it tastes like the real thing but it is a halfway crutch. It is based on coltsfoot and one of the first beneficial side-effects you'll experience from smoking this herb is the coughing up of quantities of heavy mucus and congealed waste because it is a tonic expectorant.

Even if you don't smoke, check the quality of the air you breathe, and if it is full of other people's smoke, object! I do, very strongly. I had a house-warming party where the only two guests who smoked had to stand outside on the lawn having a surreptitious drag. It is now common knowledge that passive smoking, whether it be in childhood or adulthood, greatly increases the risk of lung cancer as well as ischaemic heart disease, nasal sinus cancer and brain tumour. Cases have been recorded (in Poland) of nicotine intoxication among newborn babies breast-fed by mothers smoking cigarettes. Everyone agrees on the correlation between lower birth weight and the number of cigarettes smoked daily by the mother to be, but not many people realize that if she works an eight-hour day with someone who smokes thirty a day she herself will have passively inhaled the equivalent of five cigarettes, which is certainly enough to affect the foetus.

THE AIR YOU BREATHE
If you can, avoid areas with a high pollen count and polluted air – for example the hearts of cities, where the poisons are often dangerously high. Use an ionizer to control the balance of ions (tiny electrical particles) in the air around you. An ionizer is particularly useful in the bedroom, where you usually spend at least eight out of every twenty-four hours. You can leave windows open or closed while they are in use. Either way, they will cope. In America positive ionizers are available but in this country only negative ones are on sale. However these are almost as good although they do tend to attract stubborn dirt and plaster it to the surfaces which surround the ionizer. (For a supplier see the Appendix.)

A DIET FOR CLEANSING THE LUNGS
Don't block up your lungs with catarrh-forming foods. These include dairy products; eggs; meat; sugar; tea and coffee;

chocolate; anything refined; the gluten in wheat, oats, rye and barley; and potatoes, swedes, turnips and parsnips and any other starchy root vegetables. Include plenty of sprouted fenugreek in your diet as well as nettles, kelp, onions and garlic, the last two raw if at all possible as neither is as effective if cooked. Alternatively use oil or syrup of garlic.

Oil of garlic

Press 8 oz (225 g) of peeled, minced garlic into a wide-mouthed jar and barely cover it with olive oil. Close the jar tightly and leave it to stand in a warm place for three days. Shake it several times daily. After three days, press and strain it through a piece of muslin or fine cotton and store the resulting oil of garlic in a cool place in well-stoppered bottles.

Take 1 teaspoon of the oil hourly for colds, 'flu, and chest infections.

Syrup of garlic

Put 1 lb (450 g) of peeled, minced garlic in a wide-mouthed 4 pint (2.25 litre) jar and almost fill it with equal quantities of apple cider vinegar and plain spring water. Cover and let it stand in a warm place for four days, shaking a few times a day. Add 1 cup of glycerine and stir well. Let it stand another day. Strain and, squeezing hard, filter the mixture through a muslin cloth. Add a cupful of thin honey and stir well until thoroughly mixed. Bottle and store in a cool place.

Take 1 tablespoon three times daily before meals for coughs, colds, bronchial congestion and sore throats.

Make sure you eat plenty of vitamins A and D to strengthen and desensitize your internal mucosa. Massage blocked or inflamed sinuses with fresh lemon juice externally, rubbing it into the skin. Sinuses can also be helped by chewing freshly grated horseradish root macerated in cider vinegar. Chew a teaspoonful before each meal and when you are grating it breathe in the fumes as deeply as you can. Have a box of tissues on stand-by because the horseradish will flush out blocked sinuses very effectively. A single drop of aniseed oil on the back of the tongue will not only thrill your taste-buds, once they have got over the shock, but act as jet propulsion to clean infected sinuses.

HERBS TO HELP THE LUNGS

Herbal steam bath to decongest and strengthen the lungs

Mix ½ oz (15 g) wormwood and ½ oz (15 g) eucalyptus together. Put this mixture into a basin and pour 2 pints (1.25 litres) of freshly boiled water over it. Crush 2 cloves garlic and stir these in well. Measure in 5 drops of thyme oil. Now cover your head with a towel and hold your face 8 in (20 cm) away from this infusion. Keep the eyes closed and breathe in and out steadily through the nose ensuring that the mouth is closed. Do this for twenty minutes if you can and try to repeat it three times a day. You can use the same mixture three times over, reheating it and adding freshly crushed garlic each time.

Fennel oil used as a herbal steam bath will vaporize mucus, loosening it and causing it to degenerate so that the eliminatory process can remove it through the bloodstream far more easily than can be done by coughing, sneezing or blowing the nose. This process is helped by fennel's high mineral content. So if you don't want to go to the trouble of the elaborate herbal steam bath described above, use 10 drops of fennel oil instead added to 1 pint (600 ml) of freshly boiled water.

There is an arsenal of herbs to strengthen and help the lungs. Mullein, comfrey, sweet marjoram, elecampane, lobelia, valerian, ginseng, camomile, eucalyptus, myrrh, grindelia, nettles, coltsfoot, hyssop, horehound, angelica, elderberries, rosemary, ground ivy, Irish moss, liquorice, vervain, Iceland moss, thyme, marshmallow, lungwort, sage and, of course, garlic. It is best to drink mild herb teas like coltsfoot, elecampane, nettle or mullein daily as a prophylactic, to favour the onion family, to use horseradish as a seasoning, and to reserve the rest for use in treating colds, coughs and other occasional lung problems – because some will act as respiratory stimulants, others as relaxants and demulcents, and much depends on what's wrong with you. You may need grindelia to relax the cilia lining bronchial tubes which have become clogged up with infected mucus, or you may be better off with elecampane, which forces the lungs to give up even more carbon dioxide and so stimulates them to work efficiently. A qualified medical herbalist will help you here.

The Liver

When I explained once to a patient the function of the liver she leaned back and sighed, 'I'd rather pilot Concorde without any flying lessons than be a liver.' An astute observation. The functions of the liver are so vital that they can be likened to the activity of chlorophyll in plants. The liver is crucial biologically and is involved, in one way or another, in all the body's physiological processes. It is responsible for the secretion of bile, the formation of blood, metabolic processes, detoxification and the production of heat. The good news is that it has an amazing capacity to regenerate itself. The bad news is that it can be damaged for a long time before its great functional reserves are pushed so hard that its deterioration is detected. This is one area in which iridology comes into its own, in evaluating the exact degree of liver degeneration, and sadly most modern livers are run down and in need of help simply because they have to handle such huge burdens of chemicals and other noxious wastes including alcohol, cigarettes, coffee, allopathic drugs, radiation, air pollution and imitation food. Livers don't react too well to emotional distress either. It upsets their metabolic function.

The simplest way of decongesting the liver is to drink dandelion coffee made from dandelion root and nothing else (see Chapter 1). Dandelion root is an exceptional hepatic and acts on the kidneys too. The leaves work in the same way but less effectively.

HOW TO DO A LIVER CLEANSE
Spring is a singularly appropriate time to do a liver cleanse, after a winter of heavy body-warming foods and not enough exercise.

Ensure that your diet is light in protein (not more than 1 oz/30 g daily) and rich in raw foods and whole grains and seeds.

On rising mix 4 tablespoons olive oil with 8 tablespoons freshly squeezed lemon or orange juice and 3 crushed cloves of garlic. Save the pips from the fruit. Wallop this cocktail back quickly. It is not as horrendous as it sounds. Sip a small glass of fresh orange juice while you prepare a decoction (see Chapter 6) of fennel, liquorice and aniseed tea, the herbs to be mixed in equal parts. Drink this sweetened if you prefer. Then chew the lemon or orange pips that you have saved for at least quarter of an hour before swallowing them. Their bitter essence will stimulate the liver. Do not eat any breakfast. If you are going to work or want to be sociable, chew a clove. It will help to mask the odour of garlic. At mid-morning eat any fresh fruit of your choice.

Do this every day for two weeks and on the seventh day of each week apply a castor oil poultice (see Chapter 6) to the liver before midday and leave it on for 1½ hours. If you can, fast on carrot juice and beetroot juice on this day and take a chicory enema (see Chapter 6), using a decoction of the root, morning and evening.

Your faeces may produce a bit of green colouring during this cleanse. If you get constipated raise the amount of garlic and liquorice. If you have high blood pressure omit the liquorice altogether. If you get diarrhoea also omit the liquorice, and your mid-morning snack should be millet porridge well laced with powdered cinnamon and sweetened with honey.

A DIET FOR THE LIVER

Avoid all processed, fried and fatty foods including all dairy products. Ensure that you have plenty of vitamins A and D and calcium to assist the liver to maintain healthy internal mucosa. Take alcohol in moderation, and preferably take none at all if the liver is badly in need of regeneration. Eat plenty of anything from the onion family daily and add 2 tablespoons of lecithin granules to your diet daily.

Liver maintenance tea

    2 parts dandelion root
    2 parts agrimony leaves
    2 parts meadow-sweet
    1 part wild yam root
    1 part fennel
    1 part ginger
    1 part gentian

Drink one wineglassful of this decoction before every meal.

The Skin

The skin is your third kidney. Its hundreds of thousands of sweat glands both regulate the body's temperature, and act as miniature kidneys, working to detoxify organs and cleanse the blood. Indeed, the constituents of sweat are almost the same as those of urine. When the skin is not functioning properly its pores become choked up with vast numbers of dead cells, and uric acid and other waste gets trapped in the body, forcing the liver and kidneys to work doubly hard. Inevitably there will come a time when they can't stand the strain and start to break down and dump poisons and waste into the tissues.

Each of us should shed a pound of waste products daily through the skin but most of us manage only a few ounces. Yet the skin is the body's biggest eliminative organ and when it is working well it throws out one third of the body's waste. Certain nutrients can be absorbed through the skin, for example nutrients in sea-water and sea-air, and of course we manufacture our own vitamin D when the skin is exposed to a reasonable degree of sunshine. Heat on the skin also activates the lymphatic and blood circulation, encouraging a good flushing out of sweat from the lymph nodes.

HOW TO HELP YOUR SKIN

1. Take regular exercise involving profuse sweating. The sweat you excrete from exercise contains far more toxic waste the sweat you flush out in a Turkish bath or sauna (but these do help too, so don't neglect them – though neither treatment should be taken if you have high blood pressure or are pregnant).
2. Wear only natural fabrics next to the skin. Synthetics suffocate it. The healthiest fabric is cotton; failing that, your clothes should be of linen, silk or wool. The palms of the hands and soles of the feet are particularly richly endowed with sweat glands so don't suffocate these areas with nylon socks and non-leather shoes. Hands and feet respond particularly well to hand- and foot-baths using sweat-promoting herbs like mustard, cayenne, catnip, yarrow or lemon balm (see page 119).
3. I don't approve of the routine use of soap all over the body, but I have no objection (as some people have) to its use on sweaty or exposed parts. Choose an organic not a detergent soap. Molo and Weleda make good ones. A good alternative for cleansing the skin is soapwort. A decoction of the root yields a

lot of mucilage which looks like soapy water and cleanses skin very effectively. Fumitory and marshmallow are alternative herbal soaps but are not quite as effective. (See Chapter 4 for skin scrubs.)

4. Don't put anything on the skin you are not prepared to put in your mouth. Remember the skin is a two-way street: it flushes outwards and ingests inwards. A few drops of essential oil mixed in a carrier base of almond oil and added to bath water will act therapeutically on the skin as well as moisturizing it. Do not use mineral oil (sometimes sold as baby oil) or products containing it (as most commercial cleansing creams do).

5. Don't use deodorants. If you smell it is because your body is offloading some particularly foul-smelling poisons and you need to look to the inside not the outside to remedy the problem. I am beginning to notice, when I do an iridology test, how many women's skins are chronically blocked under the armpits because they have been stopping the natural sweating in these areas either completely with antiperspirants or partially with deodorants. Both destroy the skin's natural bacteria and upset its delicate protective pH balance. I no longer have need of deodorants. Washing twice a day should keep you smelling sweet. If you haven't reached this happy stage yet the simple solution is to wash more often.

6. Don't wash your clothes with detergents with added enzymes. In some people the body's defence mechanisms respond to enzymes by launching an assault as if it were attacking an infection. Days, months or even years later you may, if you are one of these people, develop a skin irritation.

7. The only powder designed for a low-temperature wash which does not contain enzymes is Hit Cool Wash manufactured by Camille Simon Limited and currently sold at Waitrose. Surf, Daz and Co-op automatic don't contain enzymes but are not specifically designed for the cool wash. It is better, all in all, to use natural soap to wash your clothes rather than a detergent, though admittedly this isn't making the best use of your shiny automatic washing machine which is designed to use a low-sud detergent.

8. Help the skin to eliminate by dry brushing daily (see below).

DRY SKIN BRUSHING
The benefits of dry skin brushing can be listed as follows:

1. It removes the dead layers of skin and other impurities, allowing the pores to eliminate without obstruction.
2. It stimulates circulation, so that the blood nourishing those organs of the body which lie near the surface reaches them effectively.
3. It increases the eliminative capacity of the skin.
4. It stimulates the hormone- and oil-producing glands.
5. By stimulating the nerve endings in the skin it has a powerful rejuvenating effect on the nervous system and for this reason is particularly beneficial for anyone feeling sloathful or depressed.
6. It is a good way to stop a cold dead in its tracks when used in combination with a hot/cold shower as described later in the chapter.
7. It is an excellent way of removing cellulite. Five minutes of energetic skin scrubbing is the equivalent of twenty-five minutes of jogging or any other physical exercise as far as body tone is concerned. Obviously skin brushing does not have any aerobic effect on the body (i.e. it does not directly influence the heart by exercising it).
8. It is an extremely effective technique for stimulating the expulsion of any fresh lymphatic mucus and clearing hardened or impacted lymph nodes. When it is coupled with a colon cleanse (see page 67), lymph mucus in the stool, jelly-like and ranging in colour from practically clear through honey to dark brown.
9. It helps to prevent premature ageing and induces a wonderful sense of well-being. Many of my patients complain about a lot of the things I ask them to do but I have never yet encountered one who has complained about skin scrubbing. Once they get used to it they love it!

If you want to convince yourself just how effective dry skin brushing is, brush for the first time in bright sunlight and watch all those dead skin cells flying off all around you. Then take a piece of linen, dunk it in hot water and wring it out. Rub it all over your newly brushed skin and hang it out to dry. Smell it several hours later and it will smell odd. Repeat the experiment with the same piece of linen for a few consecutive days and the reek that comes from it will surely convince you just how much dead waste is loosened by skin brushing.

HOW TO SKIN-BRUSH

Begin by buying a *natural* bristle brush with a long handle. They are not easy to come by; I import for my patients brushes made of Mexican Tampico fibre which does not gouge and scratch the skin. Avoid brushes made with nylon or synthetic fibre. Normal loofahs will not do either. (It takes twenty to thirty minutes of loofah scrubbing daily to get the effect you can achieve with just five minutes of skin scrubbing.)

Your body should be dry. Begin with the soles of your feet. Vigorously pass the dry brush over the whole of the skin except the face and genital area. You may need to avoid the nipples too if they are sensitive. Use clean, sweeping strokes, not rotary, scrubbing or back-and-forth motions. Generally, strokes below the heart should be upwards and those above downwards. Brush across the top of the shoulders and upper back for better skin contact, but if you can get someone else to do it for you they can brush from the top of the shoulders downwards towards the shoulder blades. Then they can move the brush upwards across the buttocks to meet at the shoulder blades. Pay particular attention to the soles of your feet and the palms of your hands, which are packed with nerve endings and particularly benefit from dry skin brushing.

Begin with light pressure until your skin gets used to it, then gradually as the days go by increase the pressure and the number of brush strokes over one area to a maximum of five. Brush until your skin is rosy and glowing. That is the sign to stop. When you start, brush at least once daily. The minimum should be a five-minute brush. You can also skin-scrub at night but not too near bedtime or you won't sleep.

Brush every day for three months, then brush only three or four days weekly and keep juggling these days around. So one week it may be Monday, Wednesday and Friday and the next week you may choose Sunday, Tuesday, Wednesday and Saturday, for example. The idea is to surprise your skin. Skin brushing is subject, as is the use of herbs, to homoeostatic resistance – that is, your skin will get used to it and stop responding so well.

Never brush skin that is irritated, damaged or infected. Go round it. Do not allow the rest of your family to share your brush, for obvious hygienic reasons.

You can also brush the scalp to stimulate hair growth and get rid of dandruff and other impurities. Do this working from your forehead backwards to the nape of your neck. If your hair is very long you may find it easier to massage the scalp with the flat of the fingertips, but make sure that you use an action which actually moves the scalp's skin, rather than a shampooing action.

Ideally, after a brush, you should remove the debris you have stirred up by showering. Stand in a hot shower for three minutes followed by a cold one for twenty seconds. Revert to a hot shower and then the cold, extending the time of the latter. Always move the shower head from your feet upwards, never the other way around. Finish by holding the shower over the medulla oblongata, that little organ tucked into the base of the brain which acts as a breathing pacemaker, sending out regular messages to the muscles of the chest and diaphram telling them to squeeze and relax their grip. You will find it behind a dent where the base of the skull curves inwards to meet the neck. Hold the shower here, letting it run down forcefully over your spine. When you start breathing hard it means that the medulla oblongata is thoroughly stimulated and your body has had enough. The hot–cold shower technique will alkalinize the blood and clear the head, and has a very beneficial effect on the vital functions of the body, particularly on the glandular system. If you haven't got time for a shower, rub yourself briefly all over, covering every area with a piece of wet linen wrung out.

Wash your brush in warm water, using a natural soap, once fortnightly. Rinse it well under cool running water, then shake (don't towel) it dry, and leave it in the airing cupboard to dry out completely.

HERBS TO HELP THE SKIN

The herbs which help the skin are those which purify and build the blood and support the kidneys. Fenugreek is particularly effective as far as skin cleansing is concerned. Drink six wine-glasses of the tea daily and expect to smell slightly curryfied as it works its way through the skin. Diaphoretics (preparations for inducing sweat) can be used, *but only with discrimination and caution* as they are inappropriate for many conditions. A gentle diaphoretic tea can be made with catnip or lemon balm. More powerful diaphoretics like elderflower, yarrow, peppermint, cayenne, ginger root, boneset, hyssop, pleurisy root, blessed thistle, and mustard are useful for sweating out illnesses like serious colds or fevers.

Read the sections on poultices, formentations and water treatments (see Chaper 6) as all these act directly on the skin to stimulate and heal it. Remember that skin problems are almost always the outer reflection of internal problems so do not treat them in isolation without considering the other eliminative channels.

The Kidneys

One of my best teachers used to say that he had never seen a healthy pair of kidneys, as observed in an iridology test, which I don't find surprising considering the amount of tea, coffee, cocoa, salt, alcohol and other harmful substances with which we assault our kidneys daily. Indeed I remember seeing coloured photographs of kidneys (from autopsies carried out in Germany) which had long been assaulted by huge amounts of salt and beer. The kidneys looked like the delicate shreds of coral and I wondered how they managed to function at all.

The work of the kidneys is to filter off impurities from the blood and balance the amount of salt and water retained by the body. They are located at the back wall of the abdomen right up near the ribs and, from the inner side of each kidney, a tube, the ureter, traces a path at the back of the abdominal cavity as it enters the bladder. Its exit, called the urethra, reaches an opening in the front of the vagina in women and at the tip of penis in men. In women it is shorter than in men, which is why we are more prone to cystitis – bacteria invade this short length more easily.

Most of our body is water. We eliminate about 1 gallon (4.5 litres) of water every day through the skin, the kidneys and other eliminative organs. We need an exact mechanism for controlling overall body water content, notably because even a tiny increase in the bloodstream will lead to a disproportionate increase in blood pressure. When your doctor prescribes chemical diuretics to reduce blood pressure it is because if the water content of the body can be made to reduce by as little as 2 per cent, the systolic reading can drop by anything between twenty to thirty points. Diuretics are also used to get rid of waterlogging in the body. If your ankles look like tree-trunks and your feet spill over the edges of your shoes it is a sure sign that your kidneys aren't working as they should. All chemical diuretics work by irritating the delicate tubules in the kidneys, forcing them to pass all water and in doing so they leach potassium from the body to such an extent that synthetic potassium has to be given. This begins the 'knock-on' effect of allopathic medicine, where further medication has to be prescribed to deal with the side-effects of the original drug.

Herbal diuretics all contain potassium and the various complex nutrients needed to maintain an efficient input and output. They raise both potassium and sodium levels so that the cellular pump-action improves both ways. Celery, for example, is high in sodium and has a touch of potassium while dandelion is high in potassium with a little sodium. Some herbs do irritate the kidneys, so I always advise the use of a demulcent – by which I mean herbs which are rich in mucilage and so have softening, protective and soothing actions when taken internally. Such herbs include comfrey, marshmallow, slippery elm or fenugreek taken in proportions of 20 per cent demulcent to 80 per cent diuretic. Good diuretics include agrimony, almonds, ash, burdock, buchu, birch, broom, blackcurrant leaves, bramble, briar, cleavers, couch-grass, dog's-tooth, dandelion, hawthorn, heather, horsetail, juniper, maize tassels, marshmallow, meadow-sweet, nettle, parsley, plantain, pellitory of the wall, rose, summer savoury, sage, uva-ursi, strawberry, raspberry, and redcurrant leaves. Hay-fever sufferers should not take pellitory of the wall as it may lead to allergic rhinitis. Cleavers should not be used by diabetics. Juniper needs to be used with caution; it is particularly powerful and should be used only for initial emergency treatment for cystitis. Broom should not be used by those with heart problems.

If you have to get up to urinate several times in the night it means that your nervous system is still jangling rather than that your bladder is too full. During the day, when you are mainly upright, fluid wastes drain downhill, but at night the excretion rate of the kidneys is reduced because you are horizontal. Try sleeping sitting up and you will get horrible puffy ankles for precisely this reason. After a fourteen-hour overnight coach journey in Turkey it took three days for my feet to shrink back to their normal size, and this in spite of my trying to prop them up a bit on the seat in front of me. You will need to be completely horizontal to slow the drainage down.

Never ignore a full bladder. I am continually surprised by how seldom many of my patients urinate. By holding on, the lining of the bladder gets intensely irritable as its contents are subjected to chemical change if harboured too long. A full bladder will press down on all the pelvic organs, especially the lower bowel and reproductive organs, and aggravate the possibility of prolapse.

It is unwise to treat yourself for urinary infection or kidney stones without first seeking the advice of a medical herbalist because clumsy self-help may aggravate the condition.

A DIET FOR THE KIDNEYS

Kidneys need to be flushed out, so drink lots of purified water and potassium-rich broth made from the tough outer green leaves of vegetables. Also drink fruit and vegetable juices, but avoid tea, coffee, cocoa and salt absolutely, focusing on a diet rich in fresh fruit and vegetables, low in animal products and free of all processed food. Strawberries are especially helpful as they help to dispel uric acid, and the only vegetables and fruit you have to avoid are spinach and rhubarb, which contain large quantities of oxalic acid. This can be neutralized by cooking the fruit in milk but really I don't think it is worth the trouble. If the kidneys are weak, keep your intake of water moderate as it tends to overburden them. Water-logged kidneys are evidenced by dark circles under the eyes or bagginess in this region. In this case take a herbal diuretic. A gentle and palatable one can be made by mixing 1 oz (30 g) of anise seed with 2 oz (60 g) each of dried melon seeds and dried cucumber seeds. Grind them all together in a meat mincer and mix to a paste with honey. Eat a teaspoon of the mixture with each meal.

REMOVING KIDNEY STONES

I would prefer you to do this under the supervision of a medical herbalist initially, before you go on by yourself to repeat it twice a year for prevention or maintenance, as it is quite a vigorous treatment. It cleans out the calcareous type of stone, which responds particularly well to certain herbs. The physical signs of these stones are heaviness in the stomach, an inflated belly, and yellowness or traces of red in the urine, and if a small stone moves into the ureter and jams you'll know about it – the pain is excruciating! Often X-rays fail to pinpoint kidney stones. You can help yourself by following the general advice of the diet for the kidneys and aim to drink about 3 litres (5 pints) of bottled water a day. Choose one low in mineral content.

Hydrangea root actually helps to prevent the formation of stones in excretory passages and will dissolve calcareous stones. It is also diuretic, which is vital if the fluid ingested is to be efficiently flushed through the kidneys in order to flush out stones.

Soak 2 oz (60 g) hydrangea root in apple juice (an organic one such as Aspall's is best) for three days at room temperature, shaking several times daily. On the fourth day bring the mixture to a slow simmer while covered, then set aside. One the fifth day begin a three-day apple-juice fast and having strained your decoction take 1 fl oz (30 ml) each waking hour with your juice or water until you have finished it.

Apply a poultice (see Chapter 6) of parsley with a tablespoon of glycerine added over the kidneys for at least an hour every day of the fast. This will relieve any painful congestion and accelerate healing.

Then take the following kidney formula for four months, drinking a breakfast-cupful of the decoction each morning and evening.

Equal parts of:

cayenne
ginger
golden-seal
gravel root
juniper berries
marshmallow root
parsley root
uva-ursi

Also take 100 mg vitamin B_6 and 300 mg magnesium daily. Repeat the cleanse again after six months.

CLEANSING THE KIDNEYS

Once a year in the spring or late summer it is a good idea to embark on a three-day kidney-cleansing fast. In the spring, May is the best time, as the asparagus tips are just coming through. Mince the raw green tips, catching the juice in a bowl. Take a tablespoon of juice every four hours diluted in water and drink nothing but purified water, and carrot juice mixed with equal parts of celery juice and cucumber juice. Apply a hot ginger fomentation (see Chapter 6) for one hour daily over the lower trunk so that it embraces the kidneys and the bladder. Do not be disturbed if your urine comes out smelling of motor oil. This is supposed to happen.

If you choose September, eat nothing but water-melon, including the seeds, which should be well chewed. If you can't chew them liquidize them first, but you must get them down. Follow the instructions for the poultice above.

Barley water

This is an ideal drink to soothe and cleanse the kidneys, maintaining them in peak condition. It has the added bonus of strengthening the nails and improving the quality and quantity of milk in lactating mothers, as well as helping to relieve asthma because of the hordein it contains.

Pour 1½ pints (900 ml) water over 1 oz (30 g) wholegrain barley (pearl barley won't do) and boil until the quantity is reduced by half. Add the zest rind (i.e. not the white pith) of a lemon for flavour and sweeten with a little honey or apple juice if desired. Drink freely at room temperature.

The Bowel

Everyone has their favourite hobby-horse and bowel cleansing is mine. The bowel should dump literally pounds of waste every day. Most people get rid only 8–10 oz (225–300 g) and think they are doing well if they have one or even three bowel movements daily but in truth you should be eliminating four-fifths of the food you ingest over a 10–18 hour period. You could conduct a rather novel experiment to find out if this is so by liquidizing your entire intake of food for a day, taking a long hard look at it and seeing if

most of this emerges the other end. At the same time check to see
how long food takes to pass through the body. It is not uncommon for people to retain faeces for days. You can do this with the
sunflower seed test. Eat a heaped handful of sunflower seeds,
chewing as little as possible (the only instance in which I'll let you
get away with poor chewing!) and time their passage through the
colon. They will show up very clearly, white and grey, in the
faeces. Sunflower seeds are high in vitamin F, which helps to
rebuild the mucous lining of the colon, so eat them plentifully,
and under ordinary circumstances chew them well. A sluggish
colon is just as dangerous as an impacted one. Transit time isn't
solely reliant on peristalsis (the automatic wave-like movements
of the alimentary canal by which food is propelled along it).
Much depends on the condition of the nervous system, the liver,
adrenals, pancreas and thyroid. The prolonged retention of faeces
can be one of the sources of heart disease because a poisonous
bloodstream raises serum cholesterol alarmingly, predisposing
the body to coronary disease. The biochemical changes produced
by retention may also be responsible for tumours and cancer.

EMOTIONAL INFLUENCES ON PERISTALSIS
Some people hold their tension in the neck, jaw or shoulders. I
hold mine in my abdomen and this is true of many people.
Emotional tightness, rigidity, too much control and self-
righteousness will often make the colon seize up altogether and in
this instance it is not the laxative herbs that are needed but those
that will strengthen and calm the nervous system. I find valerian
and lady's-slipper particularly helpful. Take equal parts of the
powdered herb. If the condition is chronic take one size 'O'
capsule hourly with plenty of liquid; otherwise take three capsules with each meal.

GRAVITY AND THE COLON
The other ever-present factor that will influence peristalsis is the
downward pull of gravity. The softest tissue in the abdomen is the
transverse colon and it is the only organ in the body that runs
across it completely from right to left. Prolapse of this part of the
colon is very common (and easily detected by an iridology test). A
prolapsed colon will push down on the bladder causing urination
problems. It will push down on the uterus or the fallopian tubes

or ovaries. In extreme cases an egg from the ovary is unable to pass through into the uterus, causing sterility.

One of the purposes of the colon is to flush out water from the last of the food as it passes through and if the transverse colon has collapsed and is congested the poisonous by-product of retained faeces will flood out onto the ovaries causing ovarian cysts. Women who consult me about gynaecological problems are astonished to find that their cause often lies in bowel problems (which sometimes explains why gynaecologists who just concentrate on their reproductive organs are having so little success).

Anal and rectal problems like haemorrhoids are often caused by a prolapsed colon and can be greatly eased by learning to defecate properly. Ideally you should squat with your feet flat on the floor, your knees spread and your elbows resting on them – fine if you are using a hole in the ground in France but dangerous if you try to squat on a toilet seat. Our so called 'civilized' toilets are the worst possible devices for a healthy colon, necessitating pushing down against the rectum and positively encouraging haemorrhoids. Do what I do and keep a huge pile of magazines in the toilet, not for reading but for putting your feet up on. Have the pile high enough in front of the toilet to raise your feet 6 in (15 cm) below the toilet-seat level. You will tilt back a little so rest your hands on your knees to right yourself. If all this sounds like too much palaver, simply place your hands on your head as you defecate. This will relieve the bearing down on the rectal muscles. It is not as good as squatting but it's the next best thing.

SLANT-BOARD EXERCISES

A slant board is simply a strong piece of wood big enough to lie on and positioned so that one end is supported several inches off the floor. You lie with your head at the lower end. Begin with a 3 in (7.5 cm) slope but increase this gradually as you get used to it to about 2 ft (60 cm).

These exercises will help to correct prolapsus whether it be of the uterus, stomach, colon or bladder, and they are also useful for eye, ear and sinus problems (or indeed any inflammation in the head). They are also very refreshing if you feel fatigued and muzzy-headed providing this is not the result of high blood pressure. I have a slant board in my clinic used mainly for demonstration purposes but I am occasionally to be found in the middle of a tiring afternoon lying down on it myself. It works wonders.

Caution: Slant boards should not be used by those suffering from hypertension or stomach ulcers, by those with a tendency to haemorrhage, by those with TB, appendicitis or abdominal cancer, or during a particularly heavy period.

1. With your head at the lower end of the slant board, breathe in slowly, raise your arms and stretch them above your head, reaching right back so that you touch the floor with the back of your hands behind you. When you get there breathe out and hold for a few seconds. Now breathe in again and bring your arms back. Rest them by your sides. Repeat this ten times.
2. With your arms by your sides, breathe out fully and suck your stomach muscles in so that you feel as if your abdomen is touching your spine. Hold for a few seconds and snap out, at which point you will automatically breathe in again. Relax. Repeat ten times.
3. Give yourself a stomach massage following the path of the colon from right to left (*not* left to right as for the stomach massage on page 71), or if this is initially too strenuous try rolling a small ball (about the size of a tennis ball) over your lower colon, pressing deeply as you follow its path in a big clockwise circle.
4. Holding on to the sides of the board firmly with your hands, slowly bend your knees so that they are resting on your chest. Don't worry if you can't do this fully at first – it will come in time. Now turn your head from side to side (five times to each side) while holding this position. Then, if you can, lift your head slightly and rotate it, first clockwise, then anticlockwise (three times each way), then slowly replace your legs so that they are lying flat on the board.
5. Lift your legs vertically. You can bend your knees slightly if this makes it easier. Rotate one foot outwards in a circle ten times, repeat with the other foot, then both together.
6. You will need to rest after the last exercise because it is quite strenuous. When you have got your breath back, lift your legs up again, this time keeping them as straight as you can at the knees. Bring them up to a vertical position both together. You

may need to grip onto the board hard with the sides of your hands to support yourself. Now lower your legs slowly back to the board. Repeat four times.

7. Cycle with your legs in the air working up to twenty-five times as a maximum.

8. Now relax and as you get your breath back squeeze all the muscles in your face hard, then let them go; as you do so you will feel the tension flooding from your face. As your breathing slows down to normal, feel the tension seeping out of your body. It sometimes helps to imagine it draining out of the top of your head. Rest and relax for a minimum of five minutes, letting the recharged blood circulate into your head. Get up slowly.

Another useful remedy for prolapsed organs in the pelvis is a cold sitz bath (see page 122) taken on rising. Build up to five minutes gradually. Continue daily for a minimum of three months.

COMING IN AND GOING OUT

Most people think that what they see in the toilet is what they ate a couple of meals back. In fact the normal twentieth-century diet ensures that a lot gets left behind in the colon and doesn't come out at all. Sticky refined starches that haven't been digested properly by the pancreatic secretions, drugs and barium meal as well as catarrh-forming foods like dairy products, sugar and eggs get stuck and pasted onto the sides of the colon, turning it into encrusted mucus the weight of which often forces the wall of the colon outwards to form diverticular pockets. In some people this encrusted waste can cause the colon to weigh as much as 40 lb (18 kg) and to balloon out from the customary 4 in (10 cm) to as much as 9 in (23 cm).

All this decay is an ideal home for parasites. Worms outrank even cancer as the human race's deadliest enemy and a few years ago it was estimated that some 2,000 million people were infected worldwide. One in four people in the world are infected with round-worms and autopsies reveal that 80 per cent of the people they are performed on have parasitical infestation. These parasites range in size from microscopic single-celled creatures to 24 ft (7.3 m) tapeworms. Some of my patients on a thorough bowel cleanse are quite stunned to see worms coming out of themselves, never having displayed the usual symptoms of anal irritation, dry lips during the day and wet at night, or a little pool of spit dribbled on the pillow at night – all of which are signs of worms. Worms love areas in the colon where there is little oxygen, like the caecum which colonic irrigation theory christens 'the region of worms'.

As well as tapeworms and round-worms there are hook-worms and whiplike worms, all floating about in a variety of unpleasant places and eager to crawl into a comforting and nourishing body. You can ingest them by eating unwashed food that has been grown in soil fertilized with manure that has not been properly composted. Soil in China is fertilized with human excreta and when having a colonic administered after my return from China I was not surprised to witness two quite large worms beating a hasty retreat from my colon. Tapeworms are acquired from poorly prepared pork (no wonder the writers of Leviticus banned pork products – a sensible precaution in the days before refrigerators) and from uncooked gefilte fish. They are the most difficult worms to get rid of and linger in the colon, slightly lowering iron absorption year by year but rarely going far enough to be fatal. (Obviously a parasite that actually killed its host would be rather self-defeating.)

Tapeworm evacuation

Fast on nothing but garlic, pumpkin seeds and water for two days. Then take a powerful herbal laxative like senna tea with a pinch of ginger in it. Then (and I know this sound hilarious) sit on a bucket with some warmed milk in it when it is time for the bowel to empty itself. Cold air stops the tapeworm from leaving, and warm air entices it out. It is vital to ensure that the head with its digestive suckers which look like two big eyes emerges so inspect the contents of the bucket afterwards.

Worms hate garlic, onions, cranberry and pumpkin seeds and above all they hate a clean, strong colon because there is no soft, squelchy, tasty mucus for them to latch on to.

Worms can be detected reasonably easily in an iridology test, showing up as blackened dots in portions of the bowel area and are particularly prevalent in diverticular pockets, which are an ideal breeding-ground for them. I can understand why Pasteur, one of the first biologists to discover the path of such parasites, took to examining the food he was served at friends' houses with a portable microscope!

BENEFICIAL MICROLIFE

Apart from parasites there is a huge world of microlife in our intestine. Every colon holds 3–4 lb (1.5–2 kg) of resident bacteria as indigenous flora. It is composed of 300–400 different species of bacteria whose activities affect our metabolism, physiology and biochemistry in ways that are both beneficial and harmful. So vital is this intestinal metabolic activity that it even exceeds the liver in the wide range of its metabolic processes.

These micro-organisms are both indigenous and transient. The former colonize particular ecological nitches in the intestinal tract by sticking to the mucosal epithelium; the latter are ingested in food and drink and are constantly in transit from the mouth through to the anus. Together they make up nearly 40 per cent of the weight of the faeces.

The bacterioids together with coliform bacilli and *E. coli* are the putrefactive bacteria responsible for the decaying matter in the colon. They like a diet full of protein and fat which accelerates the output of undesirable metabolites like bile salts, urea, phenols, ammonia and other dietary degradation products which are all potentially harmful substances, doubly so if there is constipation or impaired detoxification by the liver. A high population of bacterioid bacteria is one of the main contributive factors in the development of all sorts of degenerative diseases like ulcerative colitis, diverticulosis, haemorrhoids and colonic cancer and most people have a ratio of 85 per cent of these potentially harmful bacteria to 15 per beneficial bacteria.

The 15 per cent beneficial bacteria are the Bifido bacteria like *Lactobacillus bulgaricus*, *Streptococcus thermophilus* and *Enterococcus*. These produce acetic, lactic and formic acid which lower the pH of the intestine, so preventing the colonization of fungus like *Candida albicans* (which causes thrush). When the percentage is better balanced, with 75 per cent of these 'goodies', peristalsis is stimulated, flushing out toxic bacterial metabolites and waste products in the faeces, so checking putrefactive bacteria.

It is quite common for the elderly, who generally have a tired, worn-out stomach lining resulting in achlorhydria (meaning the under-secretion of hydrochloric acid), to have too many of the bacterioids. Achlorhydria is also the result of consuming too much tannic acid in tea and coffee (yet another good reason to give them up) or of taking very hot or cold drinks or foods, as well of indulging in high-fat, high-protein diets which favour meat. Bifido bacteria flourish in lacto-vegetarian diets high in fibre and wholegrains.

Hypoglycaemia and diabetes, stress and sugar, all affect the amount of sugar available to the intestinal micro-organisms which in turn influence the growth and activity of sugar yeasts like the notorious *Candida albicans*.

Breast-feeding leads to a flora with a predominance of Bifido bacteria. In the process of birth the baby is exposed to micro-organisms from the mother's vagina and intestinal tract and afterwards obtains these from the environment from being handled. The bacteria which colonize the skin and the mucosal surfaces of the upper respiratory and gastrointestinal tracts make the beginning of a lifelong symbiosis between the human organism and the indigenous flora. Bottle-fed babies have a much higher density of bacterioids, clostridia and *Lactobacillus acidophilus* with few of the benign Bifido bacteria. Breast-fed babies have acidic stools with a pH ranging from 5 to 5.5 which increases their capacity to resist infection by pathogenic bacteria. Bottle-fed babies have a faecal flora closer to those of adults in its consistency and odour, with a pH of 6–7. So breast milk clearly comes out tops Bifidogenically as well as having other immunological properties. And breast-fed babies maintain a stronger component of Bifido bacteria as they grow up than their bottle-fed cousins. It seems that breast-feeding is the first and most vital Bifidogenic factor.

I have already been on my soapbox about the hidden doses of antibiotics we receive in our food. All antibiotics cause enormous quantitative and qualitative changes in the intestinal flora, creating a perfect seedbed for pathogenic micro-organisms and actively encouraging the growth of *Candida albicans*. This is why live yoghurt (which cultivates benign bacteria in the colon) is commonly prescribed alongside antibiotics in Italy.

Ions in the atmosphere affect the growth of micro-organisms. It has long been recognized that wearing nylon tights and underwear predisposes women to vaginal thrush and wearing natural-fibre fabrics like silk or cotton goes some way to alleviating this disease. This is not just because natural fabrics encourage the proper circulation of air but because of the positive ions generated by the friction characteristic of man-made materials (negative ions, on the other hand, are health-giving).

The radiation of the abdomen with gamma rays or X-rays upsets the normal microbial balance, as do sudden violent changes in the weather.

A lot of women (especially me, as I have already mentioned) hold muscular tension in the abdomen, which hinders intestinal mobility, so affecting the microbial life of the intestine. I have found massage, abdominal yogic positions and regular use of the Pilates technique (a special form of exercise) very helpful in this respect. (See the Appendix for a contact address for the Pilates technique.)

Loud continuous sounds also affect intestinal bacteria. An interesting study recently conducted on some long-suffering mice showed that exposing them to four hours of 72 decibel rock music completely altered their intestinal flora, so avoid noisy discos and prolonged rock concerts!

The profound effect that stress has on intestinal ecology is a fascinating one. It doesn't matter where the stress comes from; the stress response stimulates the release of adrenaline and cortisol as the body alerts itself for 'fight or flight'. These hormones induce a number of physiological changes, including the drying up of oral and gastric secretions, the retention of sodium chloride and the acceleration of potassium excretion, and raised blood sugar. All these reactions change the intestinal habitat, decreasing the micro-organic goodies and increasing the baddies. When you consider how much routine stress you are exposed to from bright lights, atmospheric pressure, noise, crowds and long journeys, and how much more is self-generated from fatigue, anger, anxiety, pain and fear, it makes you appreciate just how hard it is to generate the right balance of intestinal bacteria.

Finally, strong essential oils like marjoram, rosemary, sage, thyme, clove, cinnamon and mustard all inhibit the acid production of lacto-bacteria, but interestingly after a while the bacteria adapt to the bacteriostatic effect of these essential oils, so that they can produce lactic acid. This is why Indians who crunch raw chillies are not particularly deficient in lacto-bacteria.

HOW TO IMPLANT BENEFICIAL BACTERIA

So far the tale of intestinal war sounds thoroughly depressing. But it is possible to balance your intestinal ecology by eating lots of live yoghurt daily, by which I mean 12 oz (350 g). Anything added to the yoghurt except a ripe banana will destroy much of the benign bacteria in it, so it must be eaten plain. Bananas, provided they are well ripened (and the way to tell is to choose those with brown freckles on their skins), are the only fruit known to actively encourage the growth of beneficial flora in the colon.

The problem with both bananas and yoghurt for some people is that they create a lot of mucus and 12 oz (350 g) yoghurt is quite a lot to get through in one sitting. The alternative is to take acidophilus in the form of one of two products called respectively Superdophilus and Probion. There are many other forms of acidophilus on the market but I have found these two infinitely superior in my own clinical practice. (For further details, see the Appendix.)

Either one of these, if taken in the correct dose, will exert an anti-fungal effect on the intestines. This is particularly important when you consider how *Candida albicans* produces mycelia, a network of roots which penetrate the mucosa, breaking down its function as an effective barrier. With food allergy, eczema, cirrhosis and acne there is a clear defect in the intestinal mucosa. Superdophilus and Probion also have a strong imunogenic effect, increasing the number of leucocytes and the activity of both thymus and spleen. They help correct both constipation and diarrhoea, and soothe irritable bowel syndrome. They regulate the degradation products of nitrogen metabolism such as high uric-acid levels which cause gout; they lower cholesterol levels; improve the absorption of protein; and help with migraines and headaches which are diet-related. I particularly like to use them to reestablish healthy intestinal flora after colonics, enemas or a herbal bowel cleansing programme.

Once the Bifido bacteria are balanced, vitamins can be more effectively synthesized. The intestinal flora produce a number of B vitamins including B_1, B_2, B_3, B_5, B_6, B_{12}, folic acid and biotin, and vitamin K. The indirect benefit of this vitamin production is that the bacteria themselves, requiring vitamins for their own growth, can draw on this source of vitamins rather than compete for those ingested orally. Probion and Superdophilus increase the general resistance to infections and *Lactobacillus bulgaricus* has a direct anti-tumour effect as well as being anti-carcinogenic if taken regularly.

Most interesting of all, the metabolic activity of the faecal microflora has been shown to have a greater effect on the regulation of bowel function than the addition of dietary fibre. It is not uncommon for me to encounter patients who have been stuffing themselves to the gunnels with bran (and usually wheat bran, which I don't approve of for reasons stated on page 8) and to be achieving nothing other than an irritable bowel and lots of flatulence. Both Probion and Superdophilus improve transit time through the gastrointestinal tract, which prevents auto-intoxication ('self-poisoning').

Eli Metchnikoff, the first person to appreciate the medical benefits of fermented milk, observed, 'Not only is the auto-intoxication from the microbial poisons absorbed in cases of constipation, but microbes themselves pass through the wall of the intestine and enter the blood.'

Constipation is the hub of the mechanism in the disease process. The heart of the problem lies in the passage of toxins and micro-organisms through the intestinal wall into the body in general, causing an endless array of disturbances. When the body absorbs poisons from the waste decaying in the colon the end result is self-poisoning. Meat, fish and eggs provide the most harmful metabolites, which on entering the bloodstream create a toxic load for the cells throughout the body, in particular the liver. This self-poisoning or auto-intoxication causes fatigue, poor concentration, irritability, insomnia, headaches and muscular aches, and leads to degenerative diseases.

But the implantation of benign bacteria into the colon is really the second step in a thorough colon cleanse. It is very rarely that I begin any herbal treatment without an initial colon cleanse, and this applies even to those who have six evacuations a day, because most people who have sedentary or stressful occupations, or poor posture, or who eat the average western diet, are urgently in need of it.

LAXATIVES

Most laxatives are poisonous and merely serve to irritate the bowel, doing nothing to remove the encrusted mucus. If laxatives are used regularly, the colon becomes addicted to them and in time grows weaker from overstimulation and irritation, so that the dose of laxatives has to be increased.

DIARRHOEA

It must be remembered that the cause of diarrhoea is a substance which irritates the colon so badly that peristalsis goes into overdrive in an attempt to expel it. In some cases the build-up of old faeces trapped in the colon becomes so large that these themselves induce a state of continuous rapid peristalsis, which results in chronic diarrhoea. In other words severe constipation can show itself as diarrhoea.

WHAT IS THE IDEAL BOWEL MOVEMENT?

1. The faeces should be buoyant when passed. If they sink they are heavy with mucus.
2. They should emerge easily, all of one piece and almost immediately you sit down on the toilet. As they float they should begin to break up. If it takes you more than five minutes to complete a bowel movement you are constipated.
3. Faeces should be lightish brown in colour. If their colour resembles that of the food you have been eating (for example greenish-brown after lots of green vegetables), you haven't digested the food properly. If they look yellow or chalky you have a problem with bile secretion or the production of digestive enzymes.
4. They should not smell foul, though they will have a slight odour. If you go on a fruit fast for a week and the resulting faeces smell only of the fruit you have eaten, you can be confident that you have a clean colon.
5. They should be four-fifths as bulky as the food you have ingested and they should not be compacted.
6. They should emerge unaccompanied by foaming, gurgling, flatulence and general orchestration.

Many of my patients are hopelessly embarrassed about actually inspecting their bowel movements but this is vital if you are to ascertain the health of your colon.

HERBS TO HELP THE BOWEL

Dr Christopher's herbal combination to aid in proper bowel function

This is a unique and unbeatable formula for treating all bowel problems and is also helpful as part of the treatment for haemorrhoids. It is the aim of this formulation to restore normal bowel function, *not to create a dependence*, like most laxatives do. The combination of herbs cleanses the liver and gall-bladder, starts the bile flowing, and stimulates peristalsis so that layers of encrusted ancient mucus can gradually slough off as the bowel is rebuilt, resulting in the perfect assimilation of food. It clears out bowel pockets and diverticula, healing any inflamed areas and relaxing any areas of tension.

  1 part barberry bark
  2 parts cascara sagrada
  1 part cayenne
  1 part golden-seal
  1 part lobelia
  1 part red raspberry leaves
  1 part Turkey rhubarb root
  1 part fennel

Combine all the herbs, which should be finely powdered, and fill size 'O' gelatin capsules with them.

I cannot emphasize enough that this formula produces a very individual result and therefore the dosage must be monitored and adjusted according to individual response. As there are no two people alike in age, size or physical constitution (and people's bowels are as different as their fingerprints), you will have to regulate the dose of this formula according to your own needs. I would suggest that you begin by taking two capsules three times a day, with meals, or if you don't eat three times a day take two capsules with every meal that you do eat in order to achieve a bowel movement for every meal ingested. If you get diarrhoea cut down. If you cannot get a bowel movement then raise the dosage until you can. Some of my patients have had to take as many as fifteen capsules with each meal for the first few months of this formulation. No matter. This is exactly how it should be and simply means that the patient is chronically constipated and it is taking some time before the body releases its accumulated faecal matter. Such a person can aid the initial release by using castor-oil fomentation packs (see Chapter 6).

Note what I have just said about diarrhoea and bear in mind that this formulation is just as valuable for those with diarrhoea as it is for those with chronic constipation, as well as being appropriate for almost everyone in need of a bowel cleanse at the beginning of their initial herbal programme. People with chronic diarrhoea may further assist themselves by drinking three cups a day of equal parts of marshmallow tea and mullein tea.

The bits of encrusted mucus that emerge may look very odd. You may see nuts and seeds, which may have been lodged in the colon for months or even years; traces of barium meal (if you have ever had one); bits of what looks like rubber tyre, tree bark or coloured Vaseline jelly. Alternatively bowel movements may emerge smelling particularly foul or may emerge accompanied by a great deal of rumbling or flatulence. Don't be alarmed by any of this. *Do not* taper off the formulation so much that you lose momentum and so the continuity of this elimination. I usually find a thorough bowel cleanse takes about six months but in some cases it needs to be extended to nine months or even a year. I monitor the cleanse by photographing the iris from time to time, which is particularly exciting for many patients as they can actually see the colour of the bowel, as manifested in the iris, changing.

Combine this gastrointestinal cleansing with a diet which is totally free of mucus-forming foods especially dairy products, eggs, meat and all refined processed foods. You are wasting your efforts if you pull the mucus out from one end while you continue to put it in at the other.

To determine whether the process is at an end and your colon is perfectly clean, go on a carrot-juice and purified-water fast for a day. The resultant faeces should emerge looking bright orange-brown. If they are a mixture of brown and orange brown this means there is still some old encrusted matter emerging and the process needs to be continued. If they are completely brown it means you have got a very long way to go. Fasting for one regular day a week together with taking enemas greatly helps the bowel-cleansing process.

NB Omit the golden-seal from this formulation after two months and replace it with equal parts of wild thyme and garlic. Golden-seal destroys the B vitamins if taken long term. This formulation should not in any case be taken for longer than one year.

Herbal formula for chronic constipation

I label this affectionately my TNT formula and use it only when patients really are chronically constipated to get them off to a flying start with their bowel cleanse. It should not be used for longer than two months.

Equal parts of:

Cape aloes
senna pods
cascara sagrada
agrimony
ginger
garlic
cayenne
wild yam root
alfalfa

Combine all the herbs, which should be finely powdered, and fill size 'O' gelatin capsules with them. Take them in the same way as you would Dr Christopher's formula but begin very cautiously, even in cases of chronic constipation, as it is a much more powerful formula.

In the last few months of any bowel cleanse, taper the dose down gently and begin to rebuild the blood. There is little point in doing this sooner because the bloodstream would be too toxic to take full advantage of the herbs you would be feeding it.

Dr Christopher's blood-purifying formula

This formula contains blood-rebuilders, cleansers and astringent herbs which increase the range and power of circulation, particularly to those parts of the body which have been deficient (usually the extremities in the capillary circulation). It will remove cholesterol, kill infection and elasticize the veins while strengthening the artery walls. In this way any herbal nutrients taken will travel efficiently through the blood and lymph fluids and be properly utilized.

Equal parts of:

red clover blossoms
chaparral
liquorice root
poke root
peach bark
oregon grape root
stillingia
prickly ash bark
burdock root
buckthorn bark

All the herbs should be finely powdered and put into size 'O' gelatin capsules. Take three capsules with each meal.

If you get diarrhoea it means the colon is still in the process of eliminating all that encrusted mucus, so stop the rebuilding formula, continue with the bowel cleanse and then try again in a few weeks' time. Also drink three glasses daily of the following raw juice formulation.

Raw juice for blood purification

4 parts apple juice
1 part beetroot juice
1 part carrot juice
1 part potato juice
1 part cucumber juice
1 part nettle juice
1 part celery juice
1 part watercress juice
1 part spinach juice

If blood circulation is a problem also take 1 part of horseradish juice added to this formulation together with another part of spinach juice, and a clove of garlic added to each glass.

Remember that dry skin brushing will help your blood circulation, as will plenty of exercise. While on the blood purification programme, combine it with a 2–4 month implantation of Probion or Superdophilus (see page 64).

MASSAGE TO HELP PERISTALSIS

Do this throughout your bowel-cleansing programme every morning on waking. In many people poor diet has caused their peristaltic muscles to stop working altogether and this simple massage is designed to re-educate lazy muscles.

Lie on your back with your knees slightly bent, supporting them with a cushion underneath them. Place a cushion or a pillow behind your head and neck. Now envisage your colon in your mind's eye. It comes up the right-hand side of the abdomen, crosses from right to left at the level of your elbow when you hold your arms to your sides, and goes down the left-hand side of the abdomen. It is important to place it correctly in your mind's eye so that you don't massage it the wrong way round.

Begin deep down on the left-hand side of the abdomen, with downward pressure using the heel of your hand, gradually working up the lower colon, with pressure being exerted *downwards* all the times. Now turn the corner and work along the transverse colon from left to right pressing constantly to the *left* as you work your way along to the right corner. Turn the corner again and start on the ascending colon pressing *upwards* as you gradually work down the ascending colon.

Now go back to the left-hand side of the abdomen, this time using a different type of massage movement. Press your fingertips well into the abdomen, making small circles in a clockwise direction, and as you reach the *lowest* point of each circle increase the pressure so that it becomes almost a digging motion. Gradually work up the left-hand side of the abdomen, keeping up this movement until you reach the ribs. Repeat on the transverse colon passing from left to right in a line from elbow to elbow. Begin on the left with small clockwise circles and ensure that the pressure at the end of each circle is a leftwards dig. Keep this up as you work your way backwards to the right. Now go to work on the ascending colon with small circles where the main pressure is always *upward* while you gradually move down the right side of the abdomen pressing as deeply as possible. Now revert back to the descending colon on your left-hand side and do three deep pull strokes downwards using the heel of your hand along the route you have just come. Repeat along the transverse colon moving, *right to left* using the same pull strokes. Finish on the

Stomach Massage

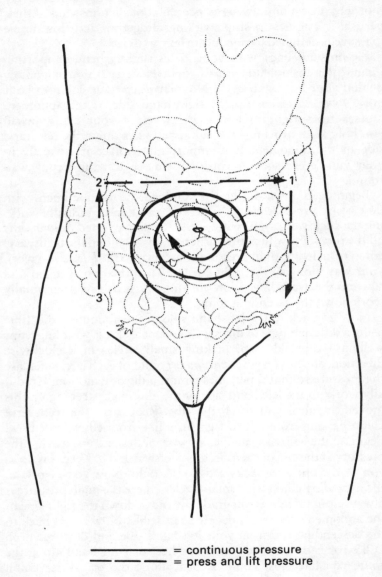

= continuous pressure
----- = press and lift pressure

ascending colon on the right-hand side, moving from the bottom to the top in the same manner.

Then move your fingers to your navel and make small clockwise circles with your fingertips using plenty of pressure. Gradually move the circular movements outwards into a spiral following a clockwise direction. When the spiral reaches out to touch the lower colon press even harder with your fingertips. Finish, spread out your palm flat just beneath your navel and give the abdomen a good hard shaking almost as if you were a terrier picking up a rat. Relax after this and rest for a few minutes as it is quite strenuous. Get up slowly. If anything hurts whilst doing this exercise ease up on the pressure a little – *but don't give up on the exercise*. Don't be put off by the lengthy instructions. It may sound complicated but if you follow the instructions step by step you will soon get the hang of it, and the results are well worth the few minutes of effort you devote to it each day.

Alternatively, there are three or four yogic positions which can be used to strengthen the walls of the colon and increase peristalsis. Ask a qualified yoga teacher about these.

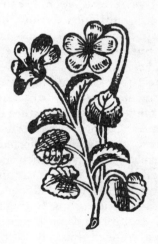

4

Beauty from the Inside Out

The Skin

By now you will be very familiar with the concept of beauty beginning from the inside out. Your skin is a reliable barometer for your overall state of health. It is the body's largest eliminative organ, weighing about 6 lb (3 kg), and far from being delicate is dynamically hardworking and, if healthy, very resilient, renewing itself with superb biochemical efficiency.

The skin is a two-way street. Not only can it push things out, it can also absorb things. Substances fed into the body can appear in the skin and those put on skin can appear in the body. Which is why it is vital to put on your skin only things you would be prepared to eat and drink.

Four factors affect the skin: environment, age, attention and genetics. Environmental assaults in terms of temperature changes, air pollutants, too little moisture or too much sun, as well as internally poor ecology in the form of poor diet, or the inefficiency of any organ, will be reflected in the skin. Some people inherit a genetic blueprint which includes translucently beautiful skin, but if they don't give it the attention it deserves it will mar that inherited treasure for their children. A brake can be put on the process of skin ageing by regular exercise, which produces thicker, stronger and more flexible skin; by regular exfoliation (removal of dead skin cells), especially as older skin tends to produce a different type of epidermis cell that does not flake off so easily when dead; by a diet like the one described in Chapter 1; by good circulation, which ensures all that nutritional goodness reaches the skin; and by sensible simple daily care.

EXFOLIATION

The finest way to exfoliate body skin is by skin scrubbing or a salt or Epsom salt rub (see page 120). The face needs to be tackled more cautiously. Men who shave exfoliate that part of their skin daily. Our alternative is to use a small stiff facial brush, a cream with abrasive particles in it or a rub-off mask. The following scrubs should not be used if you have thread veins or open lesions, but otherwise should be used two or three times weekly. For a noticeable improvement in the texture of the skin use them for five days at a stretch. Make up only a small quantity of the scrub – if the rose-petal infusion or potato is added and the scrub is left for days, it will start to rot.

Rose and oatmeal scrub (for dry and combination skins)

Choose flaky oatmeal with large, soft flakes, and mix it (adding just enough liquid to moisten the oatmeal) with an infusion of rose petals made with milk rather than water. Spread this over your face and rub the skin firmly with the flat of your fingers using small circular movements. Linger on the forehead, nose and chin. Avoid the area around the eyes. Rinse off with running warm water. Some women find it easier to incorporate the oatmeal and milk in a small muslin bag firmly tied up into a ball shape (a rubber band helps here) and then to use this as a pad to rub the skin.

Sugar, cinnamon and soapwort scrub (for spotty sallow skins)

Scrub a small potato, leaving the skin on. Then grate the potato coarsely, adding enough brown muscovado sugar to form a paste. Add 1 tablespoon coarsely chopped soapwort leaf and 1 dessert-spoon finely pulverized cinnamon stick. Mix and spread over the face. Rub the skin with the flats of the fingers, paying special attention to the spotty areas.

CLEANSING

The body's oils and waste are excreted onto the surface of the skin and are joined there by external atmospheric pollution. This motley assortment of decomposed cells, sebum, sweat, bacteria and pollutants will rapidly block the pores if it is not rigorously and regularly removed. Please note that a quick swish of soap and water will not do. In fact it may further aggravate facial debris by adding residual soap to it and leaching precious moisture from the cells, which may already be desiccated.

There are those who are utterly opposed to washing with soap at all, believing that there are better, non-alkaline ways of cleansing the skin. Perhaps at this juncture I ought to explain the whole concept of acid–alkaline balance. Normal healthy skin and hair are slightly acidic and this acidity comes from the skin's secretion. This makes up the skin's acid mantle, which protects and lubricates it. The pH (hydrogen potential) factor in any soap, shampoo or cosmetic product is the relative degree of acidity or alkalinity in that product. Some companies make soaps, shampoos and cleansers with a pH that corresponds to the acid mantle, but this ignores the fact that the pH of skin varies from person to person, and even from one part of a person to another, and at different times in the same person. Whenever the pH is artificially altered the body will return to its normal pH within a few hours unassisted and without any difficulty. The pH of the skin is measured on a scale from 0 to 14 and is generally round about 5.5. Any skin registering between 5.4 and 6.2 shows a mildly acid condition, which means that it is at its peak, well protected from infection by the acid mantle. Bacteria cannot live on an acid surface. A pH of between 6.2 and 7 means that the skin does not have enough acid and, as it is a bit alkaline, will tend to be more prone to infection. If a pH is recorded well below 5.4 the skin is too acid and will feel extremely sensitive. However, it is soap's very alkalinity which is one of the things which enables it to cleanse so thoroughly, and personally I don't feel that you can beat the lovely fresh feeling of soap and water followed by a rinse with cider vinegar diluted in fresh water (1 tablespoon to a basin of water), which will help to restore the pH balance in your skin even more quickly. Indeed I always recommend this rinse after a poultice or fomentation has been removed from the skin, or to bathe wounds.

For centuries now soap has been made from water, fatty acids, sodium salts and various oils. The modern detergent soap is really soapless because chemicals have taken the place of the various natural ingredients, but all soaps, no matter what their origin, carry out the same task of loosening dead skin cells, degreasing the skin and dislodging dirt, so that the whole mess can be rinsed away with water. I prefer glycerine-based soaps or those made with olive oil.

Provided you have not got thread veins, finish off with a cold-water splash, the icier the better. Paul Newman buries his head in a basinful of ice cubes daily and it is certainly keeping his skin (and the rest of him!) looking wonderful.

If you are still not totally convinced about using soap on your face try soapwort (see pages 46–7).

CLEANSING CREAMS AND LOTIONS

Soap won't fully remove the oil-based colours of make-up. You will need a cleansing cream or lotion which liquefies on the skin (because of the skin's warmth) to loosen and suspend the make-up debris. After tissuing it away, use a toner to remove the last of the greasy residue. By omitting the second step you will end up with only part of the proverbial horse and carriage. Without the horsepower of the toner a cleanser is useless. Nearly all commercial cleansing creams contain mineral oil – the sort of the thing which is sometimes sold as baby oil. It should not be used on you or babies as it robs the body of the fat-soluble vitamins. Choose instead natural plant or nut oils with anhydrous lanolin or beeswax as an emulsifier.

Natural preservatives

Wheatgerm oil acts as an anti-oxidant and stops creams going rank and turning dark brown. Simple tincture of benzoin (a balsamic resin extracted from trees in Java) lengthens the shelf-life of creams and lotions. Tincture of myrrh will do the same thing. Use benzoin for dry delicate skins and myrrh for oily skins. Witchhazel and apple cider vinegar will also help to preserve creams but I don't find them as effective.

As a general rule, decoctions, which have been boiled and in which most bacteria have been killed, are less likely to make creams go off than infusions (see Chapter 6). Mould starts once the cream is exposed to air, so cut out a little disc from waxed or greaseproof paper and lay this on the surface of the cream as soon as it has been potted. If you are making up a large batch keep whatever you are not currently using in the refrigerator. Don't let other people use your cream. Recent research has revealed that the bacteria passed from one person's skin to another's via the use of any communal product may cause infection.

The beauty of making your own cosmetics is that, depending on what herbs you add to them, they can be made to fulfil all sorts of functions – astringent, antiseptic, soothing or stimulating, drying or hydrating. The action of the herb can be reinforced by adding its essential oil to a decoction or infusion. Either way, the thing that really gives me personal satisfaction is the knowledge that you are only including items that are fit to eat and, this being the case, they will certainly be good enough for cherishing your priceless skin.

Lanolin

When making up a cream you have the choice of using lanolin, beeswax or cocoa butter as an emulsifier. Lanolin is quite close to the sebum the skin produces as its protective lubricant. It is also an excellent moisturizer capable of attracting moisture from the air. Your chemist will probably have two types in stock: hydrous and anhydrous. Except in cleansing creams, you will generally be using anhydrous lanolin, which has no water added. In cleansing creams, use hydrous lanolin, which will help to remove the dirt from your skin in a slurry rather than moisturizing the skin.

Glycerine

This is an excellent alternative moisturizing agent. Most glycerine is now a product of chemical synthesis and because it is no longer made from animal bones it does not involve cruelty to animals. Vegetable glycerine is available but it is extremely difficult to get hold of (for a supplier, see Appendix).

Benzoin

Two types of benzoin are made: simple and compound. Buy the simple tincture; the compound one is toxic and can hurt the skin.

Basic cream directions

The ingredients are as follows:

1. Lanolin or beeswax – 30 g (1 oz). You can amalgamate the two, varying the proportions for different consistencies. Beeswax will give your creams a stiffer, shinier consistency. Cocoa

butter can also be incorporated, mixing it with lanolin or beeswax. This will make your creams feel rich and oily. Note that some people are allergic to cocoa butter and a few to lanolin, so try a patch test (see below) first.

2. Any natural oil – 120 ml (4 fl oz). Again you can use a blend of several as long as they make up this quantity in all. I generally add about 4 teaspoons wheatgerm oil as part of my oil selection because of its marvellous healing properties as well as its anti-oxidant capacity. But it does make the cream heavier, more yellow and difficult to spread. For a less rich cream use only 90 ml (3 fl oz) of oil.

3. Any herbal infusion or decoction, or any flower water – 30 ml (1 fl oz).

4. Any essential oil from a herb or flower – 3–6 drops. The number of drops you add will depend on the strength of the essential oil and how strong you want the cream to smell. In my experience basil, bay, bergamot, clary sage, neroli, pennyroyal, peppermint, sage and spearmint are the essential oils which may in some people cause allergic reactions on the skin.

This quantity will make about 180 g (6 oz) of cream, so have a large wide-necked opaque sterilized jar standing by.

Melt the emulsifier in the top of an enamel double boiler which will stop the lanolin, beeswax or cocoa butter from burning. Now slowly add the oil a bit at a time, beating with a wooden spoon (which you should reserve for cosmetic use only) or an electrically powered whisk. Do not use a balloon whisk because it will incorporate too many air bubbles into the cream. Now remove the boiler from the stove and add the herbal water, a trickle at a time, still beating constantly. Once it is well incorporated, slow to a steady stir and keep the mixture moving until it is cooled to blood heat. Add at this point an essential oil of your choice. If you try to do so any earlier the heat of the cream will distort some of the more delicate top notes of the oil. Then spoon the mixture into your sterilized jar.

A lotion is merely a matter of varying the proportions of the ingredients. Use the same amount of emulsifier; 90 ml (3 fl oz) of any oil; 60 ml (2 fl oz) of any herbal infusion or decoction, or flower water; and 3–6 drops of essential oil.

If after a few attempts at making a cream or lotion you decide you would prefer a thicker or thinner mixture, simply vary the amount of emulsifier, oil or water. Added lanolin will make the cream thicker and tackier. More cocoa butter will make the cream thicker and oilier. More water will obviously thin the cream. More oil will thin it but will also make it much greasier.

Variations should not extend to more than 10 g (½ oz) or 20 ml (½ fl oz) either way or you will not be able to emulsify the cream. Herbs with a lot of mucilage will make the cream feel spongier.

Patch testing

Rub a little of the item you are testing onto the pulse point on your wrist, into the crook of your elbow, or into the dimple behind your ear. Use enough to cover an area about 2 cm (¾ in) square. If you are testing something that won't rub into the skin, make a paste of it by pounding it up with a little water. Let the paste dry out and then cover the area with a loose plaster of the substance with a dressing on it. Leave the patch untouched for twenty-four hours. If the skin feels perfectly comfortable and shows no sign of allergic reaction you may go ahead and use that ingredient.

HERBS FOR VARIOUS SKIN TYPES

Oily skins

comfrey (root, leaves)
fennel (leaves, seeds)
geranium leaves
horsetail
lavender
lupin seeds

marigold (petals only)
nettles
peppermint
sage
yarrow

Dry sensitive skins

borage (leaves, flowers)
house-leek
lady's-mantle
marshmallow (leaves, root)

sorrel
pansy (flowers only)
parsley
violet (leaves, flowers)

Combination skins

bay
camomile, German
(flowers only)

comfrey (root, leaves)
meadow-sweet (flowers only)

rosemary   whole rose petals
thyme

Normal skins
apple mint   lemon balm
comfrey (root, leaves)   lime flowers
cowslip (flowers)   spearmint

Just let me give you a word of warning about cowslips. I have
seen them produce in some people a condition called primula
dermatitis, which is a dark scabby eruption, the result of placing
the flower directly on the skin. By all means use the flower freely
in facial steam, teas, food and skin lotions, but don't rub it on the
skin directly.

TONING

Toners are particularly useful for getting the blood up to the
surface of the skin, which will help to nourish it, for reducing
excessive oiliness and for closing the pores. I should take the
opportunity to explain here that pores do not open and close like
doors. The words 'open' and 'close' are really a simplistic way of
describing what is a very complex physiological action. What
really happens when you apply an astringent is that an oedema is
formed round the pore, so that the skin is mildly irritated, causing
it to puff up a bit and make the pore look smaller. The effect is
soon dissipated. So skin that looks like orange peel will only ever
be temporarily redeemed.

Any herbal vinegar (an infusion made with vinegar instead of
water) makes a good toner. Choose the herb which is suitable for
your skin type. Always dilute a herbal vinegar in proportions of
1:6 with mineral water and *always* use cider vinegar for your
herbal vinegar – no other type will do. Herbal milks (infusions
made with milk instead of water) make soothing, nourishing
toners for very dry skins but they obviously go off quickly and
need to be made in small quantities and kept in the refrigerator.
Flower waters can also be used for toning and in this instance use
them neat. They are best bought. Lavender water, rose water,
orange-flower water and witch-hazel are readily available
from good chemists and elderflower water is available from
Culpeper's. Homemade flower waters are highly perishable and
are really not worth the effort.

MOISTURIZERS

Once you have grasped the concept that the outer layers of skin are dead then you will understand the necessity of moisturizing the skin. It is only the new and living cells produced deep within the epidermis that are plump and full of water. As they struggle up to the surface they lose all their moisture and emerge flattened and desiccated. Water is the *only* thing that will pump them up again, giving the skin a soft, smooth appearance. It is an excellent idea, therefore, to apply a thin layer of herbal infusion or flower water before applying a moisturizer. Simply pat a few drops onto the skin with your fingers and leave it to sink in for a few seconds only. Then spread the moisturizer on top, using it to hold the precious moisture in the skin like a piece of cling film.

Vitamin-rich skin food

    1 large raw egg yoke
    4 tablespoons apple cider vinegar
    4 capsules evening primrose oil
    1 teaspoon clear honey
    ½ cup almond oil
    3 tablespoons wheatgerm oil
    10,000 IUs oil-based vitamin A

For speed and ease make this in a liquidizer. First blend the egg yoke and half the vinegar. Now slowly trickle in half the evening primrose oil from the capsules and when it is well amalgamated add the rest of the vinegar and the honey. Finally add the rest of the oil, including the almond oil, the wheatgerm oil and the vitamin A, and store well sealed in the refrigerator.

This is an unbeatable skin food which should be used sparingly at night. (Blot off any excess with tissues as the wheatgerm oil will stain bed linen.) It is also excellent rubbed in all over after skin scrubbing and before a long hot bath. The hot water washes off any excess oil and the skin is left feeling smooth and silky. Happily the mayonnaise-like combination does not smell at all unpleasant so you won't retire feeling like a well-dressed salad! I have even used it with excellent results as a pre-shampoo conditioning pack for the hair while sitting in a Turkish bath. A shower cap stops it running down your neck.

The Hair

DIET AND THE HAIR

You must have noticed how your hair can go lank, lack-lustre and greasy within a couple of hours if you are feeling off-colour. Hair responds to a good diet startlingly quickly. Foods rich in the B-complex vitamins, or 1 tablespoon daily of brewer's yeast stirred into vegetable juice, or a generous serving of liver eaten several times weekly will all help to keep hair thick, stop it greying and prevent dandruff. Sugar, caffeine and alcohol, on the other hand, all leach B vitamins from your system. Anaemia results in brittle, wiry, thin, lack-lustre hair, but the iron to counter it is abundantly present in watercress, parsley and all dark-green leafy vegetables. Black strap molasses and yellow dock are particularly concentrated sources of iron. If taking yellow dock use two size 'O' capsules on an empty stomach morning and evening and do not neutralize its rapid effect in the bloodstream with tannin or caffeine. Iodine is particularly important for the proper functioning of the thyroid gland which in turn encourages efficient scalp circulation. All the sea vegetables are particularly rich in iodine, as is garlic. If you are taking kelp ensure that you take at least 2,000 mg daily. The effects may take three months to show, so be persistent.

Stress can play a large part in hair loss and I have treated alopecia areata (small bald patches on the scalp) in women particularly successfully using orthomolecular nutrition (medical nutritional therapy using mega doses of vitamins), nervines (herbs that are tonic and healing to the nerves), and herbs to assist the circulation and cleanse the bloodstream, together with scalp massage using essential oils of rosemary and sage and hair rinses of nettles, southernwood, marigolds and watercress.

HAIR CARE

1. Choose a brush which will move through dry hair as easily as a wide-toothed comb. Natural bristles tend to be too soft to stimulate the scalp and their closely packed formation will often tug at and damage the hair. The ideal brush has a flexible rubber base which can be easily washed, supporting well-spaced nylon bristles with uniformly rounded ends.

2. Use non-metal combs without jagged teeth which gouge and

damage your scalp. Make sure the teeth are widely spaced. Wide-toothed aluminium combs are of use only if the hair contains a lot of static electricity. They help to calm it.

3. Encourage efficient scalp circulation by massaging your scalp daily with firmly tensed fingertips. Begin at the base of your neck, working towards your forehead in small rotating circles.

4. Always protect your hair from the sun and from wind laden with salt (use a hat or scarf). Chlorine encourages the loss of iodine from the body, so if you are swimming in a chlorinated pool wear a bathing cap. If you must swim in the sea without a cap remember to rinse all the salt out of your hair as soon as you come out. Failing this, towel it dry and protect it with a scarf.

5. Avoid chemical tints, rinses, bleaches and perms. There are gentle alternative herbal methods of changing your hair colouring. Their single drawback is that the results may be less predictable.

6. Shampoo regularly with a mild herbal shampoo and always follow it with an acidified herbal rinse or conditioner. Most of us use far too much shampoo. One or two teaspoons is usually ample and I find it helpful to dilute these in a quarter of a cup of water.

   Rinse, rinse and rinse again after shampooing. It is this single factor which is my criterion for judging just how good any hairdressing salon is. Most of them do not pay enough attention to this very important step. Contrary to popular belief, it is not advisable to use a shampoo down the low end of the pH scale which is highly acid as it is possible to over-acidify your hair.

7. Never use very hot hood driers, and if you use a hand drier hold it at least 4 in (10 cm) away from the hair and move it lightly over the hair, changing its position constantly. Do not use electric curlers or electrically heated tongs.

8. Never sleep with rollers in your hair all night. Besides stretching and breaking the hair shafts and gouging the scalp you will not get a very relaxed night's sleep!

9. Never use metal-toothed rollers. Use plastic-foam or rubber ones and keep them as clean as your hair-brush and comb.

10. Use plastic-coated not rubber bands. Take advantage of all

the pretty ribbons, combs and slides currently on the market and use those instead.

11. I would like to counsel you not to perm your hair but I appreciate this is probably unrealistic, so instead I would advise you *never* to experiment with a home perm. Go to as good a hairdresser as you can. If their perm strips all the sheen out of your hair, condition it with a cup of black strap molasses, leaving this on for at least an hour – more if you can spare the time. Admittedly it is messy and it sounds extremely unlikely, but it is remarkably effective. Follow this condition with a cider vinegar rinse.

12. Do not back-comb your hair.

13. A decoction of soapwort root is an entirely natural shampoo which makes an excellent gentle hair shampoo. Fumitory or marshmallow are also useful but not quite as effective. Follow any of these with a good herbal hair rinse.

HAIR RINSES

Prepare these before shampooing, making an infusion or decoction using one or a mixture of herbs appropriate for your hair type, not forgetting at least one scented herb to make your hair smell nice. Allow the water to cool to tepid, then strain out the herbs, first through a nylon sieve and then through a coffee filter paper. This final step is especially important as it eliminates even the finest bits of herb, which you won't want left in your hair.

After thoroughly rinsing your hair with water, pour the herbal rinse through it, catching any excess in a small portable basin. Now keep pouring the herbal rinse from the basin back into your jug and through your hair again until your arms get tired. Blot the hair dry with a thick towel. Gently untangle your hair with your fingers. Do not pull it. Then use your wide-toothed comb.

HERBS FOR THE HAIR

Fair hair

camomile
cowslips
great mullein flowers
nettles
quassia bark
quince juice (extract it
    by boiling the fruit in
    water – stain, and use
    the water)
rhubarb root
turmeric

Brunettes

cherry bark
cinnamon
cloves
henna

marjoram
parsley
privet

Red hair

ginger
henna
juniper berries
marigold

red hibiscus petals
sage
witch-hazel bark

Very dark hair

elder leaves
henna
lavender
raspberry leaves

rosemary
sage
southernwood
thyme

Dry hair

burdock root
comfrey
elderflowers

marshmallow
quince blossom
sage

Oily hair

all of the mint family
horsetail
lemon balm
lavender

marigold
southernwood
witch-hazel bark
yarrow

If you are hard-pressed a dry shampoo may get you through the day but this will never equal the thorough cleansing power of a proper shampoo with water, so only use it in emergencies. The only way a dry shampoo will work successfully is to brush it out of the hair really thoroughly. Spend at least five minutes doing this. Even after the most thorough brushing, dry shampoos seem to leave some people with a dry scalp so, I repeat, use them rarely.

It is possible to obtain from some suppliers very finely powdered orris root which has a superb oil-absorbing capacity. Part the hair in sections with a comb and sprinkle on the orris root. Rub it lightly into the scalp with your fingertips. Now brush and brush and brush. Finely ground almond and finely ground oatmeal are alternatives but are not as good. White fuller's earth (not the grey, which leaves the hair looking very dingy) or finely ground corn meal may be used at a pinch.

Lavender water is excellent for very oily hair. Rose water works well for dry hair. Soak a piece of cheesecloth in one of the waters. Force the cloth over the bristles of your brush. Keep brushing through the hair. As soon as the cloth has accumulated a fair amount of oil and grime rinse it out thoroughly in water, wring it out, and repeat the process until the hair is clean and shiny.

Hot oil treatment for dry, damaged or bleached hair

1. Brush the hair vigorously, bending from the waist so that the hair and the head fall forward. Hanging over the edge of your bed is the most comfortable way to do this.
2. Heat up 30 ml (1 fl oz) of any natural oil until it is lukewarm. Add 6 drops of rosemary, lavender or basil oil to it.
3. Wet the hair well. The water will protect the hair shafts and ensure that it is the scalp that mainly absorbs the oil.
4. Part the hair in sections with a comb and apply oil to the scalp only, using a gauze or cotton pad. Massage the scalp gently with the fingertips. Pin up the the hair apart from the section you are treating, out of the way.
5. Dip a hand towel in a hot infusion (well strained) of any of the herbs recommended for oily hair. Wring out any excess moisture and wrap the towel round the head turban fashion. Cover it with a big shower-cap to trap the heat.
6. When the scalp cools repeat with a fresh hot towel.
7. Keep replacing the towels for at least an hour, two if you have the time. Do not attempt to sleep in the turban – this will only give you a crick in the neck!
8. Wash out with a herbal shampoo for dry hair. You may need two or even three shampoos to really get the oil out of the hair.
9. Rinse with copious amounts of barely tepid water and use a final rinse of any of the appropriate herbal infusions.

The Feet and Hands

One of the first things I look for as a woman walks into my clinic is what she has got on her feet and her resulting posture. Wearing shoes that fit is the foundation, quite literally, of good health. Feet are the hardest-working part of your body and contain a quarter of all the bones in the body. Leonardo da Vinci pronounced them 'the greatest engineering device in the world' yet we do tend to neglect them shamefully.

One of the surest ways I find to relax myself after a particularly trying day is to administer a foot massage. Someone else doing it for me is my idea of heaven but if you have got to go it alone here is how.

FOOT MASSAGE

Immerse your feet in soapy water or apply a herbal oil lavishly. Start by kneading the sole of one foot with your bunched fist. Now hold the foot between both hands giving a circular thumb massage all over the top and then switching this to the bottom of the foot. Now rub the ankle in a wide circular motion with your fingertips. Run your thumb firmly along each tendon on the top of the foot, working from the toes towards the ankles and at the same time squeezing the foot with a hard pumping action between your hands. Massage each toe individually with a spiralling movement from the base to the tip.

FOOT BATHS

These can be made using an infusion of geranium leaves, lady's-mantle, comfrey or marshmallow. Add a dash of cider vinegar to the water. After soaking your feet treat them to a generous rub with any of the creams you would use for your hands. Cold feet can be warmed by a dash of cayenne pepper diluted with a little talc sprinkled in the socks or better still by immersing your feet in a basinful of cold water immediately on rising for thirty seconds. Then take your feet out and place them on a towel next to the basin and spend a few minutes pretending you are picking up marbles or pencils with your toes. This really gets the circulation moving and warms your feet (although the first dip in an uninviting basin of cold water requires a bit of courage – especially first thing in the morning!). This reaps excellent results if it is practised faithfully for at least sixty days.

ATHLETE'S FOOT

This is a fungal ringworm infection causing the feet to itch, become unusually moist and smell very unpleasant. The pH of the foot changes from its normal acid balance to an alkaline one. Cider vinegar foot baths will correct this. Use soapwort not soap to wash the feet, keeping them scrupulously clean and absolutely dry. Let as much air and sun get to the feet as possible and be considerate about walking round barefoot in public places because athlete's foot is highly infectious.

Herbal bath for athlete's foot

1 oz (30 g) red clover	5 pints (3 litres) water
1 oz (30 g) sage	2 teaspoons tincture of myrrh
1 oz (30 g) marigold	
1 oz (30 g) thyme	

Make a decoction of the herbs by simmering them (but not the myrrh) in the water for twenty minutes. Strain (saving the strain herbs). Allow the decoction to cool and add the myrrh just before immersing your feet. After your feet have been soaking for about ten minutes, apply the strained herbs as a poultice, spreading them thickly between the toes. An empty basin placed beneath your feet during this operation will catch the bits of poultice that drop off. Relax. Watch your favourite television programme for half an hour, then rinse your feet and dry them meticulously. Powder them with arrowroot.

You should also cleanse the bloodstream and the lymphatic system (see Chapter 3). A small amount of poke root added to one of the formulae recommended for such cleansing is particularly helpful here.

PERSPIRING FEET

If perspiration from the feet is excessive it points an accusing finger to problems with the colon, blood and lymph stream. If you try to suppress it, it will only lead to all sorts of other damage, such as skin eruptions, as the result of toxins being trapped inside the body. Perspiration can be minimized by drinking a diuretic such as lady's-mantle, couchgrass, dandelion, fennel seed, or parsley. Foot baths containing the same herbs can also be used. Sprinkling the feet with neat witch-hazel, making sure you spread your toes so that the skin between them is well doused, also helps. Allow any excessive moisture to evaporate and then pat on lots of cornstarch. Never wear heavy socks, especially those made from synthetic fibres which prime the feet for sweating. Walk around barefoot or use leather sandals as much as conveniently possible.

An iridology test will determine the internal cause of the problem and is therefore advisable.

EXTERNAL FOOT DEODORANTS
All the advice offered for perspiring feet applies here. A double-strength infusion of lovage or cleavers, or a decoction of white willow bark will act as a natural deodorant. In each case use 2 oz (60 g) of the herbs to 1 pint (600 ml) water.

FOOT EXERCISES
To strengthen your feet and arches, pretend you are picking up marbles with your toes. Or, if you lack imagination, use real marbles. Swim as much as you can. Walk barefoot on flat surfaces as often as possible. Firm sandy beaches are ideal for this. Lying with your feet propped up over your head for half an hour daily helps take the pressure off thread veins and relieves aching legs.

EXERCISE YOUR HANDS!
You may protest that your hands get quite enough exercise, but it tends to be the sort that continually overuses them in one particular position. Revitalize your hands by trying to bring all the fingertips on one hand simultaneously to the points where the finger joints meet up with the pads of the palm. Then stretch your fingers out in full extension and hold this as hard as possible for a few seconds. Relax. Now let the fingers dangle for a moment. Shake your wrists and move your hands in circular motion. Repeat the whole routine several times first on one hand and then on the other.

LIVER SPOTS

These are a problem I am often asked about and are the result of a malfunctioning, tired liver and lack of assimilation of vitamins, E, C and B$_2$. Cleanse the liver and bloodstream (see Chapter 3) and rub castor oil into the spots several times daily.

CHILBLAINS

The Romans used to stimulate their frozen limbs while manning Hadrian's Wall by flogging themselves with nettles – a somewhat radical solution for chilblains. A less painful solution would be to assist the circulation with cayenne pepper, working up to 1 level teaspoon in juice or water before each meal, and taking 500 mg rutin daily.

To soothe chilblains

Cut a leaf of house-leek lengthways and rub the exposed juicy flesh over the chilblains twice daily.

Broken chilblains

Soak them, using a light touch, in a warm infusion of marigold flowers, then cover with a poultice of the strained-out petals, keeping these in place with a bandage. A pair of thick socks helps here if the chilblains are on your feet. Such a poultice will relieve the agony of broken chilblains very quickly and accelerate their healing.

The Nails

The nail plate from which your nail grows is several millimetres below the base of the nail and takes about nine months to emerge completely, although this process slows down radically as you grow older. Nails indicate the state of your health just as clearly as the condition of your skin, eyes and hair. Pale nails with vertical ridges indicate anaemia or extreme dryness from using too many detergents. Blue nails point to inefficient circulation or not enough oxygen. If your nails are thin and constantly breaking this may indicate inadequate vitamins, minerals and protein as well as insufficient nail care and perhaps the use of metal nail manicure sets. White spots indicate a zinc deficiency.

A DIET FOR STRENGTHENING THE NAILS

Drink one wineglassful of equal parts of horsetail and comfrey tea daily. Ensure that there is plenty of calcium, kelp, B-complex vitamins, silica and magnesium in the diet. Vitamin D cures vertical ridges; folic acid and vitamin C cure hang nails (cracks in the skin along the sides of the nail) and split nails. The former are particularly painful. They can also be treated with lavish applications of a hand cream made with horsetail and iris and the tip of dry skin which develops should be cut off rather than pulled, so that damage to the surrounding skin is prevented. Two coats of fresh lemon juice applied to the nails daily helps to strengthen them externally. If you are tackling a job that involves the use of detergents put on a pair of cotton-lined gloves underneath your rubber ones.

The Teeth

To most people halitosis is a fate worse than leprosy. Food particles in the teeth do not cause bad breath in themselves but once combined with oral bacteria plaque builds up, causing periodontal disease. Of those of us over the age of thirty who still have our teeth (and one third do not) three in every four have periodontal disease. It is the world's most widespread disease, and is insidious because it is so painless, until it is well entrenched. Bleeding gums are often one of the first ominous signs. Unhappily most people tend to ignore them, putting them down to over-zealous use of the toothbrush. But periodontal disease is widespread even amongst otherwise healthy people. Constipation will cause bad breath, as will throat infections, and obviously strong-smelling foods will too.

CORRECT BRUSHING OF THE TEETH

Do not brush your teeth in a straight up-and-down movement. Use a soft brush with a small head and rounded bristles, and spread it with a little herbal toothpaste. Holding it at an angle of 45 degrees to the teeth, scrub gently. Rinse out the mouth. Now dislodge the plaque from between the teeth with dental floss. Rinse again. Finally treat your gums to a massage using small rotating circles with your fingertips.

HERBAL MOUTH RINSES

Tincture of myrrh helps to strengthen and disinfect spongy gums. A quantity of 5 ml (1 teaspoon) to one cup of water is sufficient. Alternatively, use a tincture of thyme, sage, marigold, blackberry or tormentil in the same quantity.

NATURAL TOOTH CLEANERS

Dentists now believe that ending a meal with cheese or peanuts is a more effective way of cleaning the teeth than eating carrots, celery or apples. Cheese and peanuts leave the mouth in a non-acidic condition, which is less likely to help corrosion than the acid left behind by fruit and vegetables.

Fresh sage leaves scrubbed on the teeth have been used for centuries by the Arabs. Simply pick a leaf and rub it over the teeth. Discard it as soon as it begins to get soggy and move on to a new one. Three or four leaves should be enough to polish all the teeth and make your mouth smell sweet.

Alternatively, pound equal parts of sage and fine sea salt together in a pestle and mortar and spread out the resulting greenish powder to dry in the oven on a baking sheet. This is a superb tooth powder for cleaning nicotine stains off the teeth. Whiteness and yellowness of the teeth are inherited and I am afraid it is impossible to make yellow teeth white even with the most studious care, but cheer yourself up with the thought that the darkest yellow teeth are often the most strong and decay-resistant.

Powdered orris root and powdered charcoal mixed in equal quantities make an effective toothpaste but the flavour needs to be masked with a few drops of clove oil or peppermint oil. Avoid abrasives like pumice stone or cuttlefish-bone on the teeth. Their abrasive action will gradually wear away the enamel.

5

Grow Your Own!

Some of the plants mentioned in this book come from abroad and cannot be grown in the UK (although they can certainly be purchased dried) but the majority of them can be grown in your back garden. It is better always to be totally familiar with a few herbs than vague and lost with a pantheon. Growing herbs yourself is intensely satisfying and has the special advantage that you know exactly what it is you are harvesting. It is not a good idea to trip round hedgerows picking indiscriminately, partly because the plants could have been sprayed, urinated on or covered with lead and other noxious chemicals and partly because it is an offence to dig up *any* British wild plant without the consent of the owner of the land on which it grows, but mainly because unless you are a trained botanist you may not know what you are picking. When I was at university some students on a 'food for free' kick ate hemlock root in the mistaken belief that it was wild carrot, and nearly did not live to tell the tale – a salutary warning. But if, in spite of this, you decide you must sally out into the countryside on a plant-hunting expedition, please bear in mind the Conservation of Wild Creatures and Wild Plants Act, which first placed twenty-one species of rare plants under the protection of the law in 1975. A list of these can be obtained from the Conservation Department, Royal Botanic Garden, Kew, Surrey. And arm yourself with a really accurate book on plant identification. I particularly like *Wild Flowers of Britain* by Roger Phillips (Pan Books Ltd, 1977). It is beautifully illustrated and the scale is accurate.

It is possible to grow herbs in a window-box, in the area outside a basement flat, on a patio or a roof-top, as a lawn, in a grow-bag or a strawberry pot or on three rolling acres, if you are lucky enough to have such a plot. The beauty of herbs is that they are very adaptable and easy-going. I am sausage-fingered not green-thumbed as far as plants are concerned, yet the 200 herbs in my last garden flourished in spite of me. Indeed if you are not careful a herb garden can rapidly degenerate into a glorious dereliction, everything seeded into everything else. Plants such as mint and elder that are not self-seeding will be spreading by underground runners – the variegated kind of each of these two plants is treacherously pretty and may seduce you into letting them run wild. Don't, because in one short summer you will be contending with a jungle.

It is better to begin with a little discipline and some idea of the pattern of herb-garden you want. You do not have to go to the formal extreme of a knot garden where your herbs are tightly marshalled by hedges and bordered paths, but you may want to gravel paths in-between herb beds so that you can get at them without trampling on neighbouring plants, or to edge small beds with bricks and erect something in the centre to give the patch a focal point. Bay laurel is the obvious answer and the golden-leaved bay, *Aureus*, is a good choice. As its young shoots are the most golden part of the tree it lends itself particularly well to any position where it needs to be neatly manicured. This is best done in the spring and will encourage masses of young shoots. The only problem with bays (as my despairing husband knows to his cost having given me three so far) is that they are martyrs to scale-insects and white-fly when they are groomed. A free-standing, unclipped bush is far less likely to have mildew and pest problems.

When I moved from Shropshire to Staffordshire recently I had to re-think my herb-garden completely. My first garden had rich loamy soil and was well sheltered by a wall on one side, enjoying plenty of sunshine. My current one is very steep and tiny, clinging precariously to a rocky hillside and surrounded by low, thick stone walls. So I am growing my thyme, valerian and savory on the flat tops of the walls and encouraging house-leek to root between the cracks. I am trying *hispanica* sage for a change with its elegant narrow leaves and generous flowers. I am growing fennel right up at the top of the hill, some of it the bronze kind. (The fennel grown for use as a herb is not to be confused with Florence fennel or finnochio, the bulbous aniseedy vegetable, *F. vulgare var. dulce*, or with the giant fennel of the genus *Ferula*, neither of which have the same medicinal properties as the straightforward *Foeniculum vulgare*.) No doubt if it is successful next year I will have to be extremely hard-hearted about the prolific seedlings, though I plan to plant some of the pale yellow ones among my May-flowering tulips as an effective foil. Fennel flowers are prone to aphis infestation so I will be watching for this.

I shall miss my juniper bushes but sadly there is no room for them. It is important to grow both male and female to encourage pollination. The soft kitchen herbs, like chives, mint and parsley, I am growing under my kitchen window as they will be used frequently. And this year I am being adventurous and trying the giant chive *Allium schoenoprasum sibiricum*. I anticipate seeing the first leaves in early January and later in the summer plan to eat the flower-heads too, in bud and open. Chives love being cropped and if you do so regularly they will soldier on until November, but do let them blossom in May before you begin to barber them in earnest, and split the clumps and reset them in improved soil every second year.

My golden-leaved *Origanum vulgare aureum* will obligingly form itself into a nice neat mound but because it does not like pitiless direct sunlight I have placed it near the shelter of the garden shed. All the woody herbs can survive battering by wind but most other herbs prefer the protection of a wall, hedge or fence. None of them should be planted near voracious tree roots which steal their valuable nutrients. My horseradish I have tucked away in the roughest corner of uncultivated grass. I use so much of it that one of my patients obligingly scours derelict railway cuttings for it and brings it to me by the sackful.

My mint is firmly hemmed round with slate dug deep into the soil to stop it running rampant and I plan to root it up completely every third year and plant it elsewhere to keep it happy. Spearmint and peppermint are the two most relevant mints medicinally but I also grow apple, pineapple and eau-de-Cologne mint for culinary purposes. Like mint my sorrel has to be strictly governed otherwise it runs rampant.

In the winter I am planning to cheer up the garden with lovely fluffy bushes of cotton lavender, blue rue and slow-growing *Lavandula lavata*.

I am not too precious about the lawn. I actually like to see daisies, red clover, speedwell and yarrow growing in mine. There are even herbal alternatives to a grass lawn – camomile and thyme! Both are a lot of hard work as far as weeding and watering are concerned but their fragrance is sensational. Wait until the autumn to plant either and remember to prepare your patch first by flattening it and raking in some sort of humus (peat will do beautifully). *Anthemis nobilis* is the correct camomile for lawns but it also looks good well cropped between stonework and I once saw it used most effectively on the seat part of a stone bench. There is a wide choice of creeping thyme and if you want to be really creative try mixing the shades. Take a look at the famous thyme lawn at Sissinghurst in Kent. The intermingling of pink, white and purple is sensational.

If you have got big patches of ground to cover (and what better way to cut out the weeding?) consider ivies, periwinkles, St John's wort or lady's-mantle. All will obligingly spread rapidly. If your problem is the opposite and you have only got a 12 × 4 ft (3.6 × 1.2 m) basement to spare, think about the best use of space and light. Painting walls white helps to reflect more light and saves your plants having to crane their necks sunwards. There is generally room somewhere for at least a single 2 ft tub which should be deep to house pretty climbers like jasmine, rose and honeysuckle or even a small vine. Hanging baskets will house lots of parsley, which thrives with petunias, but you need to remember to keep these plants well watered. If herbs share a window-box with each other different ones will need to appreciate the same soil and conditions. Rosemary, thyme, lavender and sage will all soldier on together without much help or water, whereas bergamot, borage and comfrey like long drinks and deep soil. Mint, woodruff, sweet-Cicely, balm, house-leek and chervil appreciate light regular watering but do not enjoy direct sunlight.

Growing Herbs in Pots and Other Containers

Any container needs to be filled with a good layer of stones, broken crocks or gravel to facilitate drainage. Don't use garden soil – it tends to encourage fungal growths and is easily waterlogged, and if it originated in a big city it may well contain high levels of lead. Instead use a well-balanced mixture such as John Innes

No 2 with an equal quantity of Levington's and a touch of bone-meal, or use one of the modern proprietary soilless composts. Renew the compost annually. Add a fortnightly tonic of liquid fertilizer such as Biohumus, Maxicrop or one made from herbs. Manicure your potted herbs and those in window-boxes often and discreetly so that the plants do not get bald patches and look unbalanced.

All of the natural fertilizers, foliage feeders and fungicides described below can be used for herbs grown indoors and it is easy, even in towns, to find patches of nettles free for the picking. But don't pick them from the edges of carparks – they will be saturated in lead. I have noticed that raspberry, blackberry, plantain, ground-ivy and self-heal have a particular affinity for lead, and if harvested from a busy roadside may contain up to 200 times their natural lead levels. Beware.

Soil

Most herbs like a light soil. I think weeding is one of the world's great time-wasters so in the spring I cover my beds with a thin layer of dampened peat (1 in/2.5 cm will do) and this keeps in moisture as well as discouraging weeds – particularly useful when I am away from home so often. A good mulch of straw, lawn mowings or even wood clippings will also do, but remember to saturate your ground heavily just before mulching.

You do not have to go mad with constant fertilizing. Remember that most herbs flourish in their natural habitat on fairly indifferent soil, particularly the hardy ones which originated from the Mediterranean. You are not growing herbs to win prizes for size, and those richest in essential oils and nutrients are often the smallest and most unprepossessing. Any fertilizer you do use should, of course, be organic.

Composts

An elder bush or birch tree is the ideal site for an organic compost heap because the excretion from their roots coupled with those from the fallen leaves speeds up fermentation, producing a nice light compost which will revitalize your soil and can also act as your spring mulch.

Aim for a heap 3 ft square and 3 ft high (90 × 90 × 90 cm) encased in walls made of brick, wooden slats, or wire mesh on corner stakes. The whole point is to let air get in, particularly underneath. Line the enclosure with straw or old newspapers to prevent the currents of air keeping the edges too cool. (As the straw or newspaper lining will rot into the heap in time, it needs to be renewed occasionally.) Remember that you will need to get at the compost too, so make sure that one side of the enclosure can be removed. Keep your compost moist but not waterlogged. A lid of old carpet or sacking helps here. If you have less space use a ready-made compost bin.

It may be a truism but you can never have enough compost. You can make it from just about anything – weeds, leaves, lawn cuttings, and left-over food (which means a special kitchen bin into which you conscientiously drop any left-over edibles including tea-bags and peelings). Spread whatever mixture of ingredients you are using 4 in (10 cm) thick and sandwich with a herbal activator such as nettles, which are crammed with nitrogen and will instantly raise the temperature of your heap; seaweed, which is rich in trace minerals; comfrey with its high nitrogen and calcium content; or yarrow, which encourages bacteria to accelerate the decomposition. Camomile will stop excessive acidification; valerian encourages phosphorus activity; tansy adds potassium. In all these instances use the leaves and/or the flowers, not the roots, and apply a generous handful of the fresh herb per layer. I find it takes about four months to make good friable compost this way.

You can, incidentally, make a good natural liquid manure by steeping any of the herbs mentioned above in a barrel of rainwater for a few weeks, and I have two such barrels in my own garden.

Natural Fungicides

Horsetail is particularly good for preventing mint rust, mildew and blackspot, and will help any herb suspected of having a root disease. Make a decoction (see Chapter 6) using 1½ oz (45 g) to

5 pints (3 litres) water and, after straining it, spray it on to the foliage until the leaves drip.

Nettles are an excellent spray against mildew, black fly, aphids and plant lice. Prepare as for horsetail but add a desertspoon of liquid soap.

Garlic powder sprinkled among newly sown seeds discourages greedy birds, as do mugwort, rue and southernwood. I mix my herb seeds with one of them (dried for a few days) before planting so that they can absorb their aroma and this stops them being eaten by underground slugs.

Seeds

There is nothing more disappointing than sowing seeds, waiting in breathless anticipation for the tender green results to peek through and finding you have bought a dud batch. To avoid disappointment, test a few in January. Take a saucer and line it with moistened blotting paper. Place ten seeds of one type on it and cover with cling film to trap in the moisture. Put the saucer in an airing cupboard (60°F/15°C is about the right temperature) and if they have not come through in three weeks throw away the parent pack. If only half came through, don't worry because most people sow too thickly initially anyway.

Most herb seeds have a three-year life but angelica must be absolutely fresh and parsley is notoriously temperamental. You can help the latter by soaking the seeds overnight in lukewarm water to soften the seed coats. Keep your seeds cool and dry. Damp will only start the germinating and then rotting, and they will dry out if they are too warm.

Seedlings

If you are nervous about nurturing from seeds, try seedlings. They are readily available by post or to personal callers, and in the Appendix I have listed suppliers I have personally dealt with and who offer an excellent service.

When your herb seedlings arrive, open them immediately and water them with a rose attachment fitted to a can or hose. They will be suffering from shock so I generally add a drop of Bach's Rescue Remedy to mine (see Appendix). Once the herb has four distinct leaves, give it a few days in a sheltered corner outdoors to get acclimatized, and then move it to an open bed. To decant the plant, soak the pot (or plastic bag) really well, let any excess water drain out and then invert it, holding it in one hand and covering the top soil with your other hand, fingers spread to allow the seedling to poke through. Squeeze the container gently until the herb with its rootlets still firmly embedded in the soil comes out in one piece. If plastic bags prove stubborn, cut and carefully peel them away. Then transplant the herb outdoors well shrouded in its native soil, leaving the bottom of the stem a good inch (2.5 cm) below the surface. Keep watering it with one of the foliage feeders in the cool of the evening until it looks well ensconced.

Cuttings

Propagation from cuttings can be carried out in the spring or autumn. Woody herbs like sage, lavender, rosemary and thyme are easily propagated in this way. Cut or pull a 6 in (15 cm) new sprout from the parent plant just below the leaf bud or stem joint so that the twig has a heel. Dip the end in a tiny bit of rooting powder and then plant the cutting at a slight angle in a narrow hole about 2 in (10 cm) deep in a half-and-half mixture of rough sand (so the rootlets have something to cling to) and peat or compost. The mixture should be firmly packed down. Cut off any leaves within 2 in (5 cm) of the bottom (your stem cutting should be about 6 in/15 cm long) and water generously. Soft-stemmed plants such as mint and balm produce roots within a week or so, while woody ones like lavender may take eight weeks. When you can see strong leaf growth they have rooted and should be transplanted to an open bed.

Layering

This is an even simpler method of propagation which works beautifully with creeping herbs like hyssop, marjoram, rosemary, sage, horehound and all the thymes. Merely take one of the still-attached branches of the parent plant and bend it gently towards the earth, anchoring it with a V-shaped piece of wire. Then water generously to encourage root growth to spread down into the soil from the tip touching the earth and after a few weeks you will see a complete new plant forming. After six weeks you can sever it from its parent plant and transplant it.

Harvesting Herbs

This is when I always feel as if all my efforts have been doubly repaid. If I am picking wild herbs I always seek the permission of the owner of the land on which they grow, and generally you will find that once they have got over their bemusement they are delighted and you will be welcomed back to the same spot the next year. I have culled herbs in all sorts of unlikely places – feverfew from the courtyard at the back of my local dry-cleaners, black walnut leaves from the regal avenue of a stately home and valerian from a castle wall.

When you pick be selective. A small quantity of the herb judiciously picked at intervals will ensure the plant's survival and the availability of the herbs next year. Never sabotage trees by picking the bark off from the trunk. It is much better carefully to remove a few small branches from the top and outer edges of the tree because the bark is more easily stripped from these than from the parent trunk. Coax wax and gum off gently with a small sharp knife. Cut stems, don't break them. Hook high branches down with a curved walking stick so that you don't break them.

Pick herbs at exactly the right time as far as you can, bearing in mind the season, the time of day and weather conditions. Not many people appreciate that the moon's gravitational pull affects the rise and fall of sap within a plant so that a herb picked on a waxing moon will contain much more sap than one picked when the moon is on the wane. Ideally herbs should be gathered in the morning once the dew has evaporated and during a spell of fine sunny weather. Do not water herbs the day before harvesting. Buds should be culled in the spring, leaves at the beginning of summer, flowers in midsummer the moment they have unfolded, and roots, berries and barks in the autumn and not later than November. You will find that some herbs, such as balm, sweet-cicely and feverfew will crop twice if cut back vigorously after the first harvesting.

The golden rule is that if you don't know what you are picking leave it alone. Purple loosestrife looks remarkably like rose-bay willow-herb, and I could name many other examples. It is also vital to appreciate that the active principles of a plant are not evenly distributed throughout. In this book, unless otherwise stated, when I talk about a herb I am talking about the leaves. Of all the plant organs, leaves and roots are generally richest in active substances. The leaf above all is where the synthesis takes place and it is chiefly here that the numerous alkaloids, heterosides and aromatic essences are housed. Sugars, glycose and vitamins are found mainly in the roots while the stem is mainly a transit organ. The reproductive organs and their separate parts in their different stages of development contain glycosides, aromatic oils and many other valuable medicinal substances.

I have a special big, flat woven basket which enables me to separate and keep track of my herbs but a big tray will do. Don't use aluminium – it taints and stains herbs. Plastic bags are only acceptable for big roots like horseradish; otherwise they suffocate the plant, trapping moisture and encouraging a mildewed, bedraggled mess.

LEAVES
These should, of course, be clean and free of insects. If they are not, spray them well with water and nettle or horsetail tea several days before you are going to pick them. Choose the younger leaves just before the flowers open when they are richest in medicinal properties. Nipping them off helps to shape the plant and encourages growth.

FLOWERS
These must be picked the moment they are open, before their precious essential oil evaporates into the air. Cut the flower-heads off directly over a drying tray, snipping off any thick stalks as these tend to prolong the drying time. Don't bruise the flowers with your fingers.

SEEDS
These need to be allowed time to ripen in the sun and should be

gathered pod and all. It is a delicate balance trying to catch them just before wind dispersal but waiting until they are truly ripe.

BARK
This should be gathered in the early spring or late autumn when it is thick and juicy with sap and its medicinal properties are at their most concentrated. Be careful to choose only very small pieces here and there and don't injure saplings.

ROOTS
These are best gathered once the top of the plant is dying down in the autumn. You will need to dig deep and lift them out carefully without bruising them. Wash them thoroughly under cold running water and snip off any little hairy rootlets with scissors. Dandelions don't have many but valerian, for example, abounds in them.

BERRIES
These should be picked when they are luscious and glossy, well before they have even thought of turning mushy.

Drying Herbs

Fresh herbs are always preferable to dried ones as their medicinal properties are stronger, particularly those embued with their essential oils, which is why I have urged you so strongly to try growing some of your own. Besides which, the fresh taste of culinary herbs is unbeatable. But when you dry a herb by removing moisture from its cellular structure you trap the principles inside and well-dried herbs are impervious to mould and disease.

You will need to have a supply of dried herbs to get you through the winter, so it is vital that the drying is done quickly and efficiently to conserve the essential oils which increase the production of white blood corpuscles and are highly effective bactericides and disinfectants. Used externally, essential oils improve the circulation and some encourage perspiration, help soothe inflammation and act as very effective rubefacients.

When drying herbs, avoid:

1. Heating – if herbs are left piled up after harvesting they will burn from the middle like a heap of lawn clippings.

2. Bruising or crushing.
3. Spreading too thickly.
4. Drying too slowly – i.e. at too low a temperature.
5. Drying too quickly – i.e. at too harsh a temperature or in full sunlight or strong wind – as this causes fading.

The general rule is to dry herbs indoors in a warm, dark, well-ventilated place. However, sphagnum moss needs outdoor sun and wind and is spoiled by artificial heat, and comfrey can be dried outdoors to begin with, to get rid of most of the moisture before it is brought inside.

The easiest way to dry herbs is on cheesecloth stretched over a wooden frame placed in an airing cupboard. Woodier herbs can be dried in small bunches hung from hooks. Catch seeds (and stop them being muddled up) by surrounding the inverted heads with a paper bag tied firmly round the stems with a string. Perforate it near the top to encourage the free circulation of air.

The oven is not a good idea except for tough barks and berries, partly because oven heat is too harsh and the temperature varies from the top to the bottom of the oven as the door must be left partially open to ensure adequate ventilation, and also because oven-dried herbs lose a third to a half of their potency compared to their equivalents dried out of doors or in the airing cupboard which lose less than a quarter. I have a convector oven which partly solves the first snag but it is still too heavy-handed, even on the lowest setting, for leaves and flowers. When using the oven for tough barks and berries, put it at the lowest setting and partly open the door – the ideal temperature is a steady 90°F (32°C).

Seeds are ready when they crack easily between the fingernails; leaves and stalks when they feel crisp and crackly; petals when they feel paper thin; berries when they shrivel up; and bark when it snaps easily.

Storing Herbs

I store my herbs in glass jars, clearly labelled and kept firmly shut away in a cupboard. Light and heat will fritter away the active principles of a herb. My pharmacy has a heavy linoleum blind which is lowered whenever work is not in progress to encase the whole room in complete darkness.

If you are storing herbs in large quantities well-made wooden boxes are ideal. Cotton and linen bags can be used, but they need to be hung up and the herbs in them inspected periodically for moths. Paper bags are easily nibbled by vermin and insects, and plastic bags encourage mildew.

Label your herbs clearly, recording the month and year in which they were harvested and whether they were dried out of doors, in the airing cupboard or in the oven (to remind you of their different potency). Record the common and Latin name of the plant, as well as the part of the herb. My teacher Dr Christopher recounts a salutory tale of an occasion when he failed to do so and drank tincture of lobelia mistaking it for apple cider vinegar. The result was some spectacular vomiting as lobelia in large quantities is a very efficient emetic.

Barks, roots and berries will keep for two years but all other herbs will need to be replaced yearly. Treat your compost heap to the residue.

Buying Herbs

A number of firms supply dried herbs of good quality as well as essential oils and often tinctures and fluid extracts. Those I list in the Appendix I have dealt with personally. They will supply in person or by mail order.

Most health food shops now sell dried herbs but many are of dubious quality and over-priced, so do check carefully. Smell the herbs first and look at their colour. The aromatic ones should still smell of their essential oils and others should retain a nice fresh 'green' smell. They should all be clearly green, not yellow or grey or mottled, unless of course you are looking at the berries, bark or flowers, in which case the closer they are to their original colour the better. If they are brown or faded they have either been badly dried or they are old. Don't buy them. Some of the herb farms in the Appendix also supply well-dried herbs that they grow themselves so write for a catalogue, enclosing a large stamped addressed envelope.

Buying prepared herbal tablets is just about acceptable, but it is far better to make your own formulations according to your own individual needs. If you feel nervous about doing this, many are available from me directly (see Appendix for address) provided you are a patient and I have had the opportunity to examine you. No responsible qualified medical herbalist will send out herbal medicines to strangers.

The reason for this is that what you think is wrong with you very often is only the symptom not the cause, and a thorough consultation will get down to the cause, so treatment is liable to be far more successful. Besides which I find that most people need active encouragement to adopt and persevere with the kinds of diet and exercise appropriate for them. Check on the cost of any consultation and its approximate duration before you go, as prices vary quite widely.

None of my formulations are written on tablets of stone. They are ones I have found particularly successful in my own practice, but it is perfectly acceptable to substitute alternative herbs if you are sure they match up very closely. If in any doubt whatsoever please consult a qualified medical herbalist.

If you are buying herbal pills, check that they don't contain synthetic chemical preservatives such as sulphur dioxide or potassium sorbate, or artificial colours, starch, sugar, lactose, cellulose, silicon dioxide, stearates or gluten. If the assistant in the shop doesn't know (and sadly most of them are clueless) write and ask the manufacturer. Don't make the mistake of assuming that they don't contain them just because the label only lists the active ingredients. Many of the additives in herbal tablets can upset the digestive tract. The range I particularly like is made by Gerard's (see Appendix).

It may be possible to show a formulation to an assistant in a health food shop and have it made up for you. Much depends on the policy of the shop. Practising medical herbalists will insist on making up a formulation of their own for you, so please don't wave this book at them and ask for a specific formula. Your formulation will be carefully tailored to cope with your condition.

Store your herbs out of the reach of children. They are, after all, powerful medicines.

6

Using Herbs for Health

All herbs growing on good soil are perfectly chemically balanced, a state which quickly becomes distorted by heating, drying and long storage. So a herb eaten raw in its natural state is undoubtedly the most potent medicine. The problem is that most medicinal herbs are so strong tasting that they are simply not palatable. That is where the various alternative methods of employing them come in. Once you have a basic understanding of these you will be well away. Follow the instructions for the different methods of preparation carefully. One process will extract one active principle from the herb while a different process will result in activating another element altogether. For example, tincture of lobelia will act as an emetic whereas an infusion of lobelia will prove mildly sedative. A weak infusion of hops will activate aromatic principles, while a double-strength infusion will exploit the bitter tonic principle, and a decoction the astringent properties.

It is also important to understand the many ways in which a herb can be administered, because often when you are really sick you are unable to swallow anything (and remember that fasting is the best medicine of all). Besides which, the external application of herbs is sometimes the most effective way to clear up an illness. The skin, for example, is an excellent avenue into the body whether it be by water, vapour, oil, ointment, poultice or fomentation.

Medicinal Herbal Teas

These are the simplest way to take herbs but contain only the water-soluble principles of the plant. However, if teas are taken regularly over a long period of time they can be extremely effective. Fresh herbs need to be gently crushed to break up the cellulose of the plant cells, so releasing the active principles. Use a stainless steel knife, your hands or a pestle and mortar. Dried herbs should be chopped or crumbled. Don't use powdered herbs unless you fancy a muddy, unappetizing soup.

Keep a teapot specially for your medicinal tea. You will notice that your ordinary pot gets stained with tannin from your ordinary tea. If you brew an iron-rich tea like yellow dock in such a pot the iron from the herb and the tannic acid from the staining will bond together to form tannate of iron, a very strong styptic which induces acute constipation and digestive problems.

The quantities for a medicinal tea are always the same unless otherwise specified – 1 oz (30 g) to 1 pint (600 ml) boiled filtered water. (Don't use water straight from a tap which is laden with chemicals; water filters are readily available from health food shops and chemists.) From this quantity you will be able to draw about 4 wineglassfuls of tea, which you should drink a cup at a time, one with each meal.

INFUSIONS
Delicate parts of the herb – the flowers and leaves – need to be gently steeped in water for twenty minutes. First warm your special china or glass teapot, then add 1 oz (30 g) of the herb (remembering that fresh herbs will take up a lot more space than dried ones even though the weight is the same) and pour into the pot 1 pint (600 ml) freshly boiled filtered water, which has been allowed to stand for thirty seconds. (Water that is actually boiling is too harsh and destroys the potency of the herb.) Stir the tea with anything that is not aluminium, then cover the pot tightly to stop the volatile oil escaping in steam. Leave to steep for twenty minutes, then strain through muslin, nylon, silver or stainless steel. If desired, add honey, maple syrup or a dash of apple or grape juice, to sweeten.

Store what you do not drink immediately in the refrigerator, in a glass jar covered with linen or muslin to allow the tea to breathe. It will keep for up to three days like this. If you see fine bubbles popping up to the surface, the tea has begun to ferment, so throw it away on your compost heap. But if you make only a pint at a time it should be finished within a day or two so this shouldn't be a problem.

DECOCTIONS

These are made with seeds, roots, bark or very tough leaves like bay leaves, all of which need rigorous processing to make them surrender their medical properties. Put 1 oz (30 g) of the herb into the bottom of a china, glass, enamel or stainless steel saucepan, cover with 1 pint (600 ml) filtered water and a tight-fitting lid and bring to the boil. Boil gently until the water is reduced by half. Strain, hold your nose and drink. When patients complain about the strong taste I am sympathetic and try to cheer them up by pointing out that in China they drink a soupy brew which is boiled for hours, with more herbs and water added to it every so often, and never strained. Having tasted such a brew personally it may be thin compensation but I assure you it is a lot worse!

All seeds, roots and bark need to be well crushed using a pestle and mortar before use. Burdock root and cinnamon only need steeping in freshly boiled water, not boiling, and valerian should be steeped in *cold* water (for twenty-four hours) to ensure that the valerianic acid and essential oils are not lost. Decoctions will stay fresh for four days and should be stored in exactly the same way as infusions. The dosage is usually 2 tablespoons with each meal.

Essential Oils

You have a guarantee of quality if you buy your essential oils from the right places and this saves a fair amount of work. Some suppliers adulterate their oils. The ones I like are listed in the Appendix. But it is not difficult to make an essential oil yourself, albeit a dilute version of the pure oil, and as it is only the aromatic ones that are generally available it is useful to be able to make other medicinal ones yourself. Pound 2 oz (60 g) of freshly picked herb (dried herbs, in this instance, won't do) with a pestle and mortar. Scrape into a wide-necked glass container and cover with 1 pint (600 ml) vegetable oil – olive, sesame or almond. Add a tablespoon of cider vinegar to assist the breaking up of the cellulose of the herb. The container should be large enough for there to be a gap at the top so that the contents can be shaken vigorously. Do this; then the jar should ideally be placed outside in strong sunlight. It should be embedded in fine sand, which attracts and holds heat for hours after the sun has disappeared. Bring the jar in at night. Shake again and store it in the airing cupboard until morning. Keep this routine up for a week, then strain the oil through muslin initially, then coffee filter paper. Bottle in dark glass and label. In the winter, the jar should be left in the airing cupboard all the time, instead of putting it out in the sun during the day.

The process can be speeded up by using artificial heat but I never find the results quite as good. Place the closed jar in a pan of freshly boiled water and keep the water below boiling point for two hours. (This will need your more-or-less constant attention.) Strain and bottle when cool.

Taken internally oils are best mixed with a little honey and hot water, and in this case take 3 drops of the oil three times daily. Externally, dilute 2 drops in a teaspoon of vegetable oil and apply to the skin.

Tinctures

Use good-quality brandy, gin or vodka. Never use wood alcohol, surgical spirit or methanol, all of which are poisonous. The final amount of alcohol is only about one third of the original amount as the herbs, which are strained out, absorb much of it. Alcohol has the advantage over water because it will extract much more of a herb's medicinal properties than water. As the resulting tincture is therefore very potent it is only administered in very small doses, usually 10 drops at a time, always diluted in water. Tinctures will keep indefinitely and are particularly useful for masking the flavour of some of the foul-tasting herbs.

Combine 4 oz (120 g) powdered or very finely chopped herb with 1 pint (600 ml) alcohol. Shake daily and strain after fourteen days. Tinctures should be started with a new moon and strained with a full moon fourteen days later – the power of the waxing moon helps extract the medicinal properties. Then strain the tincture through coffee filter paper, into a labelled bottle and cap tightly.

If you are a teetotaller and cannot face the thought of alcohol even for medicinal purposes use apple cider vinegar instead, but add a teaspoon of glycerine before bottling.

The dosage for tinctures is 1 teaspoon or 10 drops in at least 1 cup of water three times daily with meals.

Juicing Fresh Herbs

Use fresh herbs only for this and extract the juice in a juicer. Juiced herbs are particularly useful in a fast added to bland vegetable and fruit juices. They are also useful externally as compresses. The internal dosage is 1 teaspoon diluted in juice as needed. Externally, juices can be applied liberally.

Powders

This is probably the most potent and effective form of herbal medicine because the whole herb is used, not an extract, which is why I favour powders at my clinic. You can buy many herbs already powdered from Gerard's and if you are prepared to buy a kilo or more at a time you can buy them from Brome & Schimmer (see Appendix). You can powder your own by putting them through a coffee grinder with a very powerful motor but even this will not touch some of the very hard roots and barks.

GELATIN CAPSULES

These are small cylindrical capsules made of animal gelatin into which the herbs are compressed. These are available in sizes ranging from 'OO' to '4'. The size I stock is 'O', which is the correct size for an adult. To fill the capsule, separate it and press both halves firmly into the powdered herbs until each is as full as possible. Then close the capsule carefully so that one side slots into the other.

Some of my patients prefer to measure out their powdered herbs in a capsule and then tip then into a juice, yoghurt, nut-butter or sugarless jam (such as the Whole Earth varieties), trying not to wince too much at the strong taste. I encourage this as much as I can because it ensures that the herbs are properly digested, beginning with the action of the ptyalin in the saliva, and the bitter principles once tasted stir up the liver and facilitate digestion.

Take 2 or 3 size 'O' capsules right at the beginning of each meal with lots of liquid, preferably herbal tea or a fruit or vegetable juice.

Pills

These are useful when the herb cannot be finely powdered but can be roughly chopped, and for those who hate capsule-filling. Mix 1 oz (30 g) of the herbs with enough firm-set honey or melted unsalted butter to make a malleable paste (a food mixer is handy here). Divide the paste into 100 equal-sized portions by rolling it into thin sausages, then cutting it into pellets and shaping it into balls. Roll each ball in a little slippery elm, spread them on a stainless steel baking sheet and dry them out overnight in an airing cupboard. The herb to be taken as a medicine may be extended with the addition of slippery elm or carob powder as a carrier base.

Hypoglycaemics, diabetics and anyone with a pancreatic problems *should not* use honey and people trying to lose weight should avoid both butter and honey.

Take 2 or 3 pills right at the beginning of each meal with plenty of liquid.

Syrups

These are a good basis for cough mixture. To a strained decoction add a quarter of its weight in liquid honey and thicken slowly over a slow heat, stirring with a wooden spoon until the mixture turns syrupy. You will need to skim off rising scum from time to time. Decant into a labelled glass bottle. Take 1 tablespoon as needed.

Poultices

These sound very old-fashioned but they are a useful form of treatment for external lesions, for ulcers and for drawing out boils and suppurations, as well as for applying nutriment directly through the skin via the lymph and blood circulations to the tissues and organs beneath. Poultices are also a good way of softening and dispersing material that has become hardened, such as breast lumps. You will need:

1. Herbs. Fresh herbs need to be liquidized in a little water; dried ones should be macerated in a little hot water; and powdered can stay as they are.
2. Slippery elm powder, arrowroot or cornflower as a carrier base.
3. Apple cider vinegar.
4. White fine pure cotton. A very large man's handkerchief usually does beautifully, depending on the area to be treated. Gauze is also suitable.
5. Two large plates, and a large saucepan of boiling water.
6. Plastic sheeting (such as a piece of bin bag or those plastic bags that come from the dry cleaners, or cling film), stretchy cotton bandages and safety pins.

Estimate enough herbs to cover the area to be treated to a depth of ¼ in (6 mm). Mix these with about a tablespoon of the carrier base and enough apple cider vinegar to form a thick paste. Spread the piece of cotton onto a plate and put this over a saucepan of boiling water. Scrape the herbal mixture into half the cotton, keeping it from the edge to stop it squelching out when you use it. Fold the other half of the cotton over the top, then fold the damp edges together and press out any excess moisture. Cover the whole with the other plate until the poultice is really hot. Remove and apply it as hot as is bearable to the affected area, but obviously don't burn yourself. Cover with plastic; secure with bandages and safety pins or, if the area is very large, a thin towel. Leave it on all night. If the poultice is to be applied somewhere on your trunk wearing a tight cotton T-shirt will help to hold it firmly in place.

The next morning peel the poultice off and warm it up using the plate method. Meanwhile cleanse the area by bathing in a warm decoction of echinacea. Reapply the poultice but this time use the other side against the skin. Repeat each evening with a completely fresh poultice (using it again in the morning) until the area is healed.

HERBAL FORMULAE FOR POULTICES

These are listed for convenience in alphabetical order.

Breast lumps

2 parts saw palmetto
1 part poke root
1 part linseed

Burns and deep wounds

2 parts comfrey
1 part lobelia
equal quantities honey and wheatgerm oil

Mix in enough honey and wheatgerm oil to make a thick paste. This needs to be left on permanently until the area beneath is completely healed and it falls off of its own accord. Apply thickly over immobile areas, thinly over areas that move. If for any reason you have to remove it (and try to avoid this) soak it off with a warm decoction of equal parts of echinacea and goldenseal. Keep the burn out of the sun for at least a year, and as soon as the skin is strong enough skin-scrub daily (see Chapter 3).

Congestion, swelling and respiratory problems

2 parts lobelia
1 part marshmallow
1 part linseed

Drawing poison out of the skin

1 part slippery elm
1 part linseed
1 part plantain
½ part cayenne

External itching

3 parts chickweed
1 part arrowroot
1 part slippery elm

Sprains, fractures and torn muscles

1 part horsetail
1 part comfrey
1 part lobelia
1 part slippery elm

Swollen glands

3 parts mullein
1 part lobelia
1 part plantain
1 part slippery elm

MINI-POULTICES

These are useful for outdoor emergencies such as bites and stings. Pick clean leaves of plantain, marshmallow, vine, geranium or dock, and chew them rapidly to a pulp, mixing with plenty of saliva and not swallowing. Spread this directly onto the swelling, and if you have have it to hand cover with a piece of plastic or cotton to hold the mini-poultice in place until you can get indoors and do a proper job with equal parts of lobelia and slippery elm, or alternatively cayenne and plantain.

Fomentations

These are thin liquid poultices which are particularly useful if a large area has to be treated. Hot fomentations encourage the circulation of lymph or blood to a specific area, so relieving swellings like varicosity and goitre, muscular aches and colds. Cold fomentations ease head congestion, insomnia, fever, indigestion, sprains, bruises and sore throats.

I use both hot and cold fomentations a lot in my practice, and although going to bed accompanied by the rustle of bin bags may not be too romantic I do find them extremely effective, especially if used on a regular cyclical basis. As well as being made from fresh, dried or powdered herbs, all fomentations can also be made from warmed oils, expressed plant juices, tinctures and fluid extracts diluted in water.

HOT FOMENTATIONS

Make a double-strength herbal decoction or infusion, using 2 oz (60 g) herb to 1 pint (600 ml) water and strain, mashing the herbs well down in the sieve to extract every last bit of goodness from them. Powdered herbs are particularly effective in this instance. Reheat the liquid and dip into it white pure-cotton cloths (bits of old white sheet will do nicely), wringing them out lightly. Wrap them round the part to be treated and secure with bandages and cling film or a piece of some other plastic. Protect the bed sheet with towels to prevent it staining and leave the fomentation on all night.

Limbs are best treated by using long cotton gloves, fine cotton or silk stockings, or linen bandages wrapped round puttee style, secured with silk stockings or cotton tights on top. This is very effective for varicose and thread veins as well as eczema, psoriasis and ulcerous conditions. Sustain the heat over the area concerned for as long as you can with a hot-water bottle. Don't use an electric heating pad. I used to recommend this but have since grown to appreciate just how much electronic pollution we are subjected to and how damaging it can be.

COLD FOMENTATIONS

These are made in the same way as hot fomentations, but let the liquid grow cold before dipping the cloths in. A cold fomentation left on for 5–15 minutes will encourage blood to move quickly to the surface in cases of high temperature, sprains and bruises. For fever, change the fomentation every 5–10 minutes as it heats up. A cold fomentation left on for 20–30 minutes will relieve indigestion and insomnia and may be repeated, if necessary, once every two hours. A cold fomentation left on all night will relieve a sore throat and bring down swelling. It is especially effective for water on the knee.

CASTOR OIL FOMENTATIONS

These were widely used by Edgar Cayce, an American psychic, to heal many different ailments including digestive problems, Hodgkin's disease, Parkinson's disease, pelvic cellulitis, microbial infestation and kidney problems. The medicinal properties of the oil of castor beans have been recognized for thousands of years, and I sometimes find that my own patients are already familiar with the external use of the oil to clear up liver spots and to increase lactation in nursing mothers. Certainly in my own practice I have found castor oil – coupled with internal herbal help (including enemas), massage and hydrotherapy – superlative for clearing up a wide variety of digestive and reproductive problems. You will need:

1. Two pieces of white woollen flannel, both cut to double the area you intend to cover. Woollen stockings will do for the feet and thin blankets of fine wool are also acceptable.
2. A large piece of plastic of medium thickness.
3. Several hot-water bottles.
4. Bath towels.
5. Safety pins.
6. A plastic cover big enough to cover the bed or sofa.
7. A large bottle of castor oil.
8. Hot water.

Method

1. Heat up the castor oil in an enamel-lined, china or glass saucepan.
2. Immerse one piece of flannel in it and stir it round with tongs, ensuring that it gets thoroughly saturated.
3. Meanwhile cover the bed with plastic and a large bath towel to protect the sheets.
4. Lift out the saturated flannel and place it over the area to be treated. Be careful here and don't apply it so hot that it burns the skin.
5. Cover it with the duplicate piece of flannel soaked in hot water and wrung out so that it is damp but still steaming. Rubber gloves help here.
6. Now wrap the area securely in the plastic, then a towel, and secure with safety pins.
7. Lie down gingerly and pack the area being treated with hot-water bottles.
8. Leave on all night or for a minimum of 1½ hours.
9. Strip off the pack and store it in a plastic bag so that it can be reused for three or four nights consecutively. (Then rest for three nights. Then start again with a new pack.) To reuse the pack, put the oil-soaked piece of flannel back in the sauce-

pan, pour in more castor oil, and reheat the flannel, again stirring it round with tongs.

10. After taking off the pack, sit in the bath carefully and clean the skin with 2 teaspoons of bicarbonate of soda dissolved in 2 pints (1.25 litres) hot water. This will prevent any possibility of skin rashes. Don't panic if your skin is very red and blotchy. This is temporary and merely a sign of how actively the castor oil is working.

11. If treating digestive disorders, take 2 tablespoons olive oil and 1 tablespoon freshly squeezed lemon juice on the third night every week of treatment.

One of my patients healed her husband's diabetes by using this pack faithfully and consistently for six months.

Water Treatments

All herbs can be ingested into the body through the skin via osmosis, which is why applying herbs directly to the skin is so effective. Herbal baths need to be very strong to be effective and hand and foot baths work particularly well because the extremities are the most receptive parts of the body.

HAND AND FOOT BATHS

Mix a double-strength, unstrained decoction or infusion of herbs with an equal quantity of freshly boiled water, then pour it into a large (heat-proof) enamel, china or glass container. Immerse the feet in the water, which should be bearably hot, for eight minutes exactly, on rising before breakfast. Hand baths should be taken before supper for the same length of time. Continue this tailing and topping cycle for three days, reheating the mixture as you go; then throw it away and begin again. Take the baths for six days weekly, resting on the seventh day.

Epsom salt and herbal hand and foot baths

These are extremely effective for painful, swollen tendons such as are a feature of arthritis and rheumatism. Add a whole pound of Epsom salts and 1 teaspoon in all of mustard, cayenne and ginger to a washing-up bowl half full of hot water. Stir well to dissolve, then soak the hands and feet for 15–20 minutes and as you do so work each appendage well, under the water. With feet it helps to pretend you are lifting pencils with your toes. When you have finished, briefly rinse the hands or feet in cool running water and massage well with cayenne ointment.

Mustard hand and foot baths

These work wonders for aching and burning feet, leg cramps and as a preventive measure against chilblains (provided they have not yet appeared). Add 1 tablespoon mustard powder to a bucket of hot water and soak up to the knee or elbow in it for ten minutes. Massage the hands or feet afterwards with tincture of benzoin and camphor.

BATHS

Add a gallon (4.5 litres) of strained decoction or infusion to a medium-filled bath. Immerse as much as possible of the body under water for twenty minutes, resting the head on a folded towel or bath pillow. Clean the skin before you take the bath by vigorously skin-brushing and washing any really grubby bits with a non-detergent soap and/or flannel. If you use any kind of soap *after* any sweating therapy it stops the cholesterol from coming out through the pores.

Epsom salt and cider vinegar baths

This treatment is *not* to be used by those with high blood pressure or a heart condition, but it is an excellent way of dispersing acidity in the system, soaking up aches and pains, getting the skin to work properly, inducing a short fever for therapeutic purposes, and cleansing the system of fungus. It is also a good bath to take at the onset of a cold and is particularly beneficial when you are following a purification programme. In this instance take such a bath every second evening for six days, then rest on the seventh day. Put the plug in the empty bath and stand in the bath massaging yourself all over with equal quantities of Epsom salts and almond oil, using small circular movements and working towards the heart. This exfoliates dead skin. Let the salts and oil fall into the empty bath. Then step out of the tub and fill it as deeply as possible with hot water, adding an additional cup of Epsom salts and one of apple cider vinegar. Stir to dissolve. Soak yourself in the bath for at least half an hour, adding more hot water as it cools. Drink as many cups of a diaphoretic tea as you can manage. Ginger is my favourite and I usually prepare a large thermos flask in advance, but yarrow, catnip, peppermint, elder-flower and pleurisy-root will also do. These teas will encourage perspiration and the elimination of toxins. Elimination through the skin is vital. Normally the skin does one twentieth of the work of the kidneys but by speeding it up with herbs and hydrotherapy it can take on one tenth of their work, so preventing the kidneys from becoming overloaded.

Have some ice-cubes on stand-by in a bowl, together with a couple of flannels, so that you can use these on your face, neck and forehead if you feel dizzy, sick or faint. As the water drains out run a cold shower over your face and body and let it cool down thoroughly. Go to bed warmly dressed and pack yourself round with hot-water bottles to encourage free perspiration. Some of my patients sweat so prolifically that they need to get up in the middle of the night to change into fresh night-wear which is all to the good.

Do not wear any kind of body lotion after this treatment. Leave the skin to breathe freely. The next morning take a shower, and then by all means use your body oil or lotion.

TURKISH BATHS AND SAUNAS
For those with bronchial congestion or sinus problems a few drops of eucalyptus, peppermint or camphor oil mixed with the water which is dashed over the coals in a sauna is helpful. In a Turkish bath take in a small cotton cloth soaked in a few drops of the oil and hold it near your face. In both cases breathe in deeply through the nose and out through the mouth.

VAPOUR BATHS
These are particularly effective for bringing down cholesterol levels, for relieving arthritic pain and for throwing out rubbish from the system during any deep-cleansing procedure. They work well with balm of Gilead; tincture of lobelia, benzoin or myrrh; oil of wintergreen, lavender or eucalyptus; or witch-hazel. The easiest way to construct one at home is to throw a blanket across a line and sit on a low wooden stool with your head poking out of the 'tent'. Put a facial steamer (even though it is not your face that

you are steaming) inside the tent filled with water and a teaspoon of whatever herbal extract you are using and switch it on. (Facial steamers are sold in most large department stores.) The area beneath the tent will soon be filled with vaporized steam. Stay in until the steamer is empty of water. Rinse your face briefly with warm water and pat, don't rub, dry.

The American Indians used to use these therapeutic steam baths, squatting over burning stones drenched in water whilst wrapped round in blankets.

The whole procedure sounds ridiculous but, if you can take the trouble to go through with it, it is probably the most effective hydrotherapy of all.

SITZ-BATHS

These can be awkward to take but they are very rewarding, relieving pelvic congestion and facilitating circulation, so speeding the healing of the whole reproductive area. Taken cold, a sitz-bath will combat fatigue and stimulate elimination. Taken hot before bed, it will warm the body and relieve rectal complaints. Except in the instance of a shower, herbal decoctions, infusions and tinctures can be added to the water in the treatments described below as needed.

Cold sitz-baths

Fill your bath tub with 6 in (15 cm) cold water so that when you sit in it the water comes up to your naval. Now climb in, sit down and raise your feet to about the level of the water, bracing them on the end of the bath. You can always put in an up-ended plastic bucket as a foot rest if this proves too tiring. Let your knees fall apart and scoop up handfuls of water, vigorously splashing it over the abdomen while you count slowly to sixty. Wrap yourself in a towel and without drying lie down for at least ten minutes. If you feel a nice warm glow after this, gradually increase to a slow count of 180 over twelve sessions or more.

Hot sitz-baths

A hot sitz-bath can be taken before a cold sitz-bath if you are feeling chilly or to relieve the discomfort of an anal fissure or haemorrhoids. Follow the same procedure using comfortably hot water.

A sitz-bath substitute

Stand with your back to the shower so that the warm water is aimed at your lower back. Now bend over and back into the shower parting your legs so that the water runs between your buttocks, and gradually increase the temperature to the hottest you can manage. Now turn the shower onto cold and have it running forcefully while you count to forty. Once you have mastered this increase the count to eighty. Finish as for a sitz-bath.

Gargles

For maximum effectiveness these should be used as hot as possible. They can be made from infusions, decoctions and tinctures and act to relieve sore mouths and throats. A few drops of tincture of myrrh in half a cup of hot water is good for mouth ulcers, and a double-strength infusion of sage leaves with a teaspoon of cider vinegar added to each cup is excellent for sore throats including laryngitis. A cup of ginger water (a decoction made with either fresh root ginger or powdered dried ginger) with 1 teaspoon apple cider vinegar, 2 teaspoons honey, the contents of a capsule of garlic oil and a generous pinch of cayenne is a delicious mixture to gargle with and then drink, and will soothe bacterial throat infections. Tonsillitis can be helped by gargling with a teaspoon of tea-tree oil diluted in warm water.

Eye-baths

These should be made from very gentle herbs like cornflower, marigold, raspberry leaves and eyebright. Always brew them fresh, strain them meticulously several times through coffee filter paper and wash out *both* eyes, even if only one is infected, using a sterilized eye-bath and changing the wash for each eye. Alternatively apply lukewarm compresses and keep changing the wash for each eye. Alternatively apply lukewarm compresses and keep changing them as they cool.

Ointments

These are used for their protective and emollient effects and are generally made with a herbal oil and beeswax or cocoa butter combination and kept covered with wax-paper to prevent deterioration. Use a pint of herbal oil to 2 oz (60 g) melted beeswax or cocoa butter. Add essential oils only once the mixture has cooled considerably, but before it begins to set. Beeswax gives a stiff pasty consistency, cocoa butter a richer oilier one. Ointments are particularly effective for dry and cracking skin and need to be applied generously and rubbed in thoroughly.

Creams

Being lighter versions of ointments, creams are easily absorbed and are excellent for treating sore and chapped skin and protecting and moisturizing healthy skin. Their moisturizing effect is enhanced if you spray first with a flower water or diluted apple cider vinegar. (For how to make a cream see page 78).

Vaginal Douches

Douches reduce the incidence of vaginitis (which two out of every three women suffer from at some time in their lives), relieve painful periods and are essential after the use of vaginal boluses. They are a very active form of treatment, so use only mild herbs well strained, at body temperature unless otherwise directed, and never take more than two douches daily – and this only in cases of stubborn infection. Stop douching as soon as the infection clears, otherwise the delicate balance of natural bacteria in the vagina will be altered. It helps to maintain the pH balance by adding a tablespoon of apple cider vinegar or a teaspoon of fresh strained lemon juice to every 2 pints (1.25 litres) of herbal infusion or decoction. I am not too keen on plain yoghurt. It seems to cause even worse irritation with many of my patients.

Your douche kit should be scrupulously clean. (Vaginal douche kits can be bought by mail order from the address given in the Appendix.) Make an infusion or decoction (depending on the herb used) and strain through coffee filter paper. Allow to cool to body temperature. Hang the douche bag, which has a strong hook attachment, on the wall over the bath 2 ft (60 cm) above the hips. Climb into the bath and lie down. (It helps to warm the bath up first by running hot water round it then letting it drain out.) Insert the nozzle slowly and gently into the vagina so that it touches the cervix and lie back. Release the closed tap slowly, allowing the herb tea to flow into the vagina. Then using both hands close the vaginal opening against the nozzle so that the vagina literally becomes flooded. If you do this correctly you will detect a slight sensation of pressure as the vagina obligingly expands to accommodate the fluid. When it feels full, shut the tap with one hand, releasing your hold with the other and allow the vagina to drain. If you have done it properly the liquid will be rapidly expelled with a swoosh. Now repeat the whole procedure until all the tea is used up. Douching whilst sitting on the toilet or bidet is tantamount to useless. Don't bother with it.

Warning: Pregnant women should never douche, and avoid douching for at least four weeks following delivery.

Enemas

These are used to treat nervous complaints, pains and fevers; to cleanse the bowel and stimulate the detoxification of the liver, spleen, kidneys and lymph; to relieve inflammation; and to carry nourishment into the body. If women have experienced an enema at all it is usually just before childbirth and it has usually been administered amidst fear and discomfort. Often soapy water is used (which makes me tremble with anguish whenever I think about it as it wipes out all the acidophilus from the colon) and induces violent and often painful peristalsis. I am not therefore at all surprised that when I mention enemas to women most of them get very apprehensive.

Please let me reassure you. An enema is really easy and comfortable to administer. I have patients get themselves into a dreadful tangle through sheer apprehension, but if you lay everything out in advance and give yourself plenty of time and privacy you will find that taking an enema is easy, and the more relaxed you are the easier it is.

Enemas do not make a mess. Your anal sphincter muscles will hold the liquid in the colon until you decide to release it. Initially the stimulus the enema fluid gives the bowel may make you want to rush straight to the toilet and release it, but you will acquire more self-control with practice.

Taking an enema is really quite logical. No sensible person will attempt to unblock a drain from the top end of the waste-pipe. Using the same analogy, a blocked colon needs to be relieved from the bottom end. In the event of a fever, an enema is the quickest way to relieve the bowel of toxic waste. If you are so weak that you cannot eat then an enema of spirulena or slippery elm will supply some nourishment. If a colon is inflamed, as with colitis, an enema of slippery elm will soothe it and line it protectively.

You will need:

1. Herbal decoction or infusion – 3½ pints (2 litres). Cool enemas are used for cleansing, warm ones for treating nervousness and spasms. Always use plain spring water bottled in glass. *Never* use tap-water. It certainly contains chlorine which will upset the bacterial balance in the colon, and may also contain fluoride.
2. An enema kit (see Appendix).
3. Oil, Vaseline or KY jelly.
4. A large bath-towel or a piece of plastic sheeting.

Taking an enema

1. Fill up the enema bag with a strained tea (warm or cool, as appropriate) and hang it from a hook at shoulder height.
2. Lubricate the tip well with oil, Vaseline or jelly.
3. Lie down on your right side with your knees tucked up to your chest and gently press the lubricated tip of the enema tube into the rectum.
4. Release the tap and allow the liquid to flow slowly into the rectum. If it encounters a block of impacted faeces (you will know because you will feel marked internal pressure) turn off the tap, roll over onto your back with your knees bent and soles of your feet flat on the towel and massage the area in an

anticlockwise direction. Once you feel comfortable roll over onto your right side again and reopen the tap.

5. When the enema bag is emptied of its contents turn off the tap and remove the nozzle tip.
6. Wrap yourself up warmly in a bath-towel and go and lie down on a slant board (see Chapter 3).
7. Retain the enema for twenty minutes. Get up carefully and release whilst sitting on the toilet.

The smell of what comes out may be very strong and objectionable. Remember, you are releasing some old impacted matter which is tantamount to stirring up an old blocked drain, so don't be alarmed. Initially some people have a great urge to void but this is only because their bowel's elasticity is so poor. With practice they get better.

Warning: Enemas should only be taken while fasting except in emergencies when they are being used to treat fever. They should never be overused or relied on in place of a proper bowel movement.

Pessaries and Boluses

These are really just shaped internal poultices. They are made by adding enough finely powdered herbs to gently warmed cocoa butter to form a doughy paste. A vaginal bolus is then shaped into a sausage the size of a regular-sized menstrual tampon. A pessary should resemble your little finger in size, and if it is being used to treat the colon not just the rectum it should be at least 2 in (5 cm) long and two should be inserted, one behind the other. Round both ends for easy insertion.

The best way to roll out the paste is on an oiled marble slab or inside a plastic bag. The pessaries or boluses can then be left overnight on a flat plate in the refrigerator to harden, and then stored there in a sealed plastic bag, each pessary or bolus wrapped in greaseproof paper.

Once unwrapped, the pessary or bolus should be inserted as deep into the rectum or as high into the vagina as possible, just before bed. Body heat will then gently melt the cocoa butter and release the herb. The bed linen should be protected with an old towel, and you should wear cotton knickers and a press-on sanitary towel. Rinse the anus or the vagina well the next morning, preferably in a cold sitz-bath. A new pessary should be inserted after every bowel movement, a new bolus on the evening of every second day. You should douche on alternate evenings (not the evenings on which you insert a bolus) resting from both douching and the boluses or pessaries on the seventh day.

Pessaries and boluses are useful for astringing (i.e. tightening) internal tissues, soothing, cleansing, drawing out poisons and carrying herbs to the requisite area internally to treat infections, irritation, cysts, tumours and, in the case of pessaries only, haemorrhoids. Boluses and pessaries usually work well over a period of six to seven weeks. Expect all sorts of discharges and odours as they do their work.

You may need to hold a bolus in place with your fingers when you are pressing down for a bowel movement. If it keeps falling out plug it in with a homemade tampon of natural sponge which you will need to take out gently and wash morning and evening.

Love-making is perfectly comfortable if the bolus is soft and beginning to melt but it is best done after douching. Douche again afterwards and continue the cycle. Obviously if you have a vaginal infection love-making is not advisable.

Don't worry if the bolus disappears altogether never to re-emerge. This often happens and is a sign that the body is desperately in need of the nutrition of the herbs. Sometimes you may have to help the bolus out with your finger, which is easiest done squatting.

Storing Herbs

Anything made with alcohol, vinegar or glycerine will keep for at least a year if stored in an opaque, well-stoppered glass bottle. But herbal formulae, no matter how effectively dried or preserved, all grow less effective with age. In my own pharmacy the herbal powders, pessaries and boluses are made up weekly but then I see a fair number of patients. You will probably not be able to turn your stock around so quickly, so remember to throw away any dried herbs (except roots, berries and barks) once they have passed their first birthday.

Syrups will keep indefinitely as honey is an excellent preservative. Even so I would advise you to store them in the fridge. Essential oils will keep indefinitely in opaque glass bottles but air gaps should be eliminated as they are used, by transferring them to smaller and smaller jars. Poultices and fomentations should always be freshly made. Cotton bandages and sheets should be well boiled after use, dried, and stored in plastic bags. All herbal preparations should be stored in glass containers – never plastic ones, which absorb other smells and disintegrate under the influence of essential oils.

You will soon know when herbal preparations have gone off. They smell odd, fizz or turn ominous colours, in which case treat your compost heap to them. My guiding dictum is 'If in doubt throw it out.' To save yourself the expense of doing this, buy only a few ounces of the herbs you need at a time unless your family is enjoying lots of certain teas you have grown. It is better to share with a friend than to be landed with stale stocks. I know communities where one person volunteers to grow a few herbs and another some different ones, and these get shared around as needed, which seems sensible.

Cautions

HERBS FOR RESTRICTED USE
Some herbs are not to be used at all, or should not be used in certain circumstances.

Cooked spices
Most cooked spices aggravate. They are more therapeutic taken raw in capsules. This especially applies to cayenne. If you don't want to take it in capsules, or if you have a sensitive stomach mix it with vegetable juice or take it with soya milk. Cayenne may cause a burning sensation during defecation.

Golden-seal
This should not be used by diabetics as it lowers blood sugar levels. Taken over a long period of time, say three continuous

months, a patient may begin to exhibit hypoglycaemic symptoms. If this occurs, drink liquorice tea (provided there is not high blood pressure) or fenugreek tea. In the long term it will stop the assimilation of B vitamins. Golden-seal is useful in the short term and is especially effective as an infection-fighter used as a vaginal douche. Large doses contract the uterus so women who have a tendency to miscarriage should not take it.

Lobelia

This is not commonly available to the general public as it is (in my opinion erroneously) considered a poisonous herb in this country. Herbal practitioners are able to prescribe it and I often include it in my formulae as it has a wonderful way of catalysing other herbs and getting them to work in the parts of the body where they are most needed. Administered in small doses it acts as a superb antispasmodic, relieving asthma and helping to bring up mucus. One part of lobelia should always be mixed with at least three parts of another herb. In large doses it is an emetic.

Sage

Being rich in tannin it should not be used on a daily basis as tannin builds up proteins and eventually reduces the assimilation of the B vitamins. Very prolonged use of such astringent herbs have occasionally been associated with throat and stomach cells becoming cancerous, so they are all best used only in the short term. If they do have to be used for some time, mix them with milk to neutralize the tannin. Herbs high in tannin are the bark of bayberry, cascara and blackberry, the roots of comfrey, sarsaparilla and yellow dock, and some leaves like peppermint, cleavers and uva-ursi.

Sage also contains a toxic ketone as part of its essential oil complex, and if the essential oil is consumed regularly over several months, this produces an emmenagogic effect in women, causing womb spasming and the possibility of abortion in pregnant women.

Sassafras

The oil is carcinogenic, so always use the whole herbs. Do not use during pregnancy for longer than three or four consecutive weeks.

False unicorn

This contains oxytoxic agents which promote delivery and should not be used during the course of pregnancy except to resolve potential miscarriage problems (see page 185) and during the last six weeks of pregnancy (see page 187).

Red raspberry leaf

This contains fragine, which strengthens the uterus but cannot promote uterine contraction unless a woman has a genetic background of strong pelvic muscles. Its high iron content makes it useful in pregnancy but it is best administered with at least the same quantity of other herbs.

Liquorice

This decreases the contraction of the uterus and should not be taken during labour or in the last six weeks of pregnancy. Indeed, unless prescribed by a medical herbalist, it is best avoided altogether during pregnancy.

Large and frequent doses exacerbate high blood pressure because it is a cardiac stimulant with a high sodium ratio. (Most other herbs are low in sodium and high in potassium.)

Ginseng

This is best used in chronic diseases where the patient is weak, cold and debilitated. It should not be given to those with hot acute diseases, nor to those suffering from high blood pressure or nervous tension or anxiety, nor to women with menstrual irregularities. It should never be taken with anything containing caffeine. For the elderly or for prolonged treatment of debilitation take 400–800 mg of the dried root daily. The young and active should not take it for more than three weeks without a break of at least a fortnight. For short-term use take 600–2000 mg daily.

All this applies to Asiatic ginseng (Panax ginseng) and Siberian ginseng (*Eleutherococcus senticosus*), which if anything is even stronger, and to a lesser extent to American ginseng (*Panax quinquefolium*). The best way to take ginseng is using all three mixed together in equal parts. Natural Flow supply these (see Appendix).

Hawthorn berries
Do not use if you have low blood pressure.

Garlic
The whole clove eaten is very beneficial for high blood pressure but the expressed oil (in the form of garlic pearls) can sometimes aggravate the condition, so approach it with caution.

Horsetail
This is a strong diuretic and therefore its long-term use is danger-ous as it can scour the kidneys. Always use with a demulcent to soften its effect. (I generally mix it with marshmallow.) It contains silicic acid, saponins, alkaloids and a poisonous substance called thiaminase which causes symptoms of toxicity in both humans and animals. Thiaminase poisoning causes a deficiency of vitamin B, and may lead to permanent liver damage.

All diuretics need to be approached cautiously, especially juniper berries which are wonderful for clearing up cystitis but need to be used only briefly. The only really safe diuretic is dandelion root, which contains potassium in plenty but is not as potent as horsetail or juniper berries.

Aloe juice
Not to be confused with the whole herb, aloe vera, or with aloe gel, both of which are more potent in their action and should never be used internally. Externally a cut leaf rubbed over burns, rashes, psoriasis, insect bites and itching works wonders, but if you eat the whole plant it will cause ulceration and piles. The juice taken internally actually heals internal ulceration. As it may cause griping mix it with ginger juice. Aloe juice is available from G. R. Lane (see Appendix).

Lime tree flowers
Use only fresh supplies. Old fermenting leaves can cause hallucinations.

Nutmeg
This contains a poisonous alkaloid, strychnine, and should not be used at all except by qualified medical herbalists. It can cause abortion.

Camomile
Often regarded as the gentlest of herbs, overstrong infusions will cause nausea, so I generally specify that it is to be taken at half the normal infusion strength – i.e. take ½ oz (15 g) to 1 pint (600 ml) water and infuse for only ten minutes.

Nettles
Do not use the foliage in its fresh state after July as it becomes a laxative.

Violets
Always use the fresh not the dried flowers.

Aconite
The aconites belong to the *Ranunculaceae* family, of which there are between 300 and 350 species, all containing the deadly poisonous alkaloids aconitine and pseudoaconitine. If they are ingested in anything but the most microscopic quantities the results are fatal.

Belladonna
Safe only in the hands of qualified medical herbalists, this is part of the *Solanaceae* family and one of the most notorious plant poisons.

Foxglove
If taken in excess it is deadly.

Groundsel
Excessive use over short periods may cause cirrhosis of the liver.

Heart's-ease
Excessive doses may cause cardiac reaction.

Hemlock
The hemlock that Socrates drank was administered with opium because otherwise death would have come by an excruciatingly slow progressive failure of the respiratory system; the opium made this a little more bearable. Avoid also *Cicuta*, water hemlock, which is just as fatal.

Mistletoe

Government authorities are sensitive about this herb partly because of its anti-carcinogenic reputation but also because it contains large amounts of viscotoxins. Take it only under medical supervision.

Pilewort

This should never be ingested fresh or rubbed on the skin fresh – it may cause irritation. Once dried the toxins in the plant break down into the reasonably innocuous anemonine and it is safe to use.

Poke root

The leaves are extremely poisonous. It contains toxic mitogenic substances (i.e. substances that distort cell structure) and should not be taken in doses of more than 1 g every twenty-four hours, and then should only be used for six days, after which it should be given a wide berth for three months. Properly administered it is a wonderful cleanser for the lymph and blood and is excellent for chronic catarrh and benign cysts.

Clover

Some varieties of white or Dutch clover contain hydrocyanic acid, which can break down into prussic acid in the digestive system and prove extremely poisonous. New Zealand is the only country to record a death from clover poisoning but incidents of toxicity occur regularly.

Rue

If inhaled in large amounts it is hallucinogenic.

Squill

This can cause drastic diarrhoea and uncontrollable retching. It needs to be prescribed in minute, carefully monitored doses.

Tobacco

Chewed raw or taken as a tisane it causes vomiting, convulsions and respiratory failure, even in minute doses. Nor is the Italian gypsy habit of applying it as a poultice to an ulcer or wound to be recommended as it is possible that enough of the toxin could be absorbed into the bloodstream to cause poisoning.

Buttercup
The sap is extremely poisonous.

Holly
The leaves are sometimes used to treat rheumatism but the berries are poisonous.

Broom
It should not be used if there is high blood pressure or during pregnancy.

White bryony
In large doses it is toxic.

Greater celandine
Christened both the best and the most wicked of herbs, in large doses it is extremely poisonous. I use it only externally and its sale is restricted to medical herbalists.

Celery
Ascertain the source of the seed, which is usually dressed with fungicide, and only use it if you can be confident that this is not the case. As it is a uterine stimulant, it is not to be taken in pregnancy.

Valerian
Once the stress crisis is over (see page 205), substitute an alternative nervine. In the short term its action is quick and potent. In the long term it causes degeneration of the nervous system.

PHYSICAL SENSATIONS
Some herbs, such as kava-kava and cloves, will numb the tongue. Lobelia in tincture or tisane form can cause a feeling of scratchiness in the back of the throat. Bayberry bark and myrrh cause a tightening sensation in the mouth in tea or tincture form. Prickly-ash may make the stomach very hot and will produce profuse sweating. Blue cohosh applied externally is extremely irritating to the mucous membranes, as is the fresh juice of poke root. Cayenne may cause anal burning on defecation.

ESSENTIAL OILS

It takes 7,000 flowers to make one drop of undiluted essential oil so they should be treated with a great deal of respect and caution. Pennyroyal oil, for example, can easily cause a painful and dangerous abortion. Coma, bleeding, uncontrollable trembling can all occur with excessive dosage and they should be taken strictly according to instructions, dissolved in hot water with a little honey. Externally they are usually applied to the skin diluted with a mild carrier oil.

HERBS FOR SHORT-TERM USE ONLY

Golden-seal

After 2–3 months of use take it out of the formula and replace it with an alternative mixture. There is no exact substitute, but I find that a combination of equal parts of wild thyme and garlic is reasonably effective.

Poke root

Use for six days only and then not for another three months.

Black and blue cohosh

Both are potent herbs and useful in the short term. You will be warned off excessive doses by nausea.

Senna and cascara bark

Used over the long term they actually discourage peristalsis.

Sassafras, horsetail, juniper and kava-kava have all been mentioned already.

IF POISONING BY PLANTS DOES OCCUR

Induce vomiting as quickly as possible (unless the plant was taken several hours beforehand in which case vomiting is a waste of time) and then phone the doctor.

Keep the patient calm. Panic merely increases the speed with which a poison invades the system. Ipecac syrup (1½ fl oz/45 ml for an adult) will quickly induce vomiting. Lobelia (5–10 ml in peppermint tea) will also do so. Never clear up the vomit until the doctor has inspected it. Undigested plant material in the vomit can give important clues about the nature of the toxic material swallowed.

Vomiting may leave the patient feeling better, albeit rather weak. Do not assume, however, that the worst is over. Do not try to induce vomiting more than once. *All* poisoning victims need immediate professional help.

Your First Aid Kit

Accidents happen even in the best-regulated families and a well-equipped first aid cabinet is invaluable under such circumstances.

Buy small jars of chickweed or marigold ointment or make them yourself. Put any tinctures or oils in small dropper bottles and aim to stock about 1 fl oz (30 ml) of each one. Fill at least eight capsules and carry them in small, clearly labelled plastic packets, and have a few spare empty capsules at hand. Have scissors, tweezers, bandages, a thermometer, plasters, gauze and a 5 ml teaspoon on hand.

The following remedies are offered in alphabetical order of the name of the herb for convenience.

Aloe vera
Rub the juice squeezed from the leaf over sunburn and minor burns and reapply frequently. If the burn is more severe apply powdered comfrey root, wheatgerm oil and clear honey in equal parts as a poultice and leave it on. Do not attempt to peel it off. Simply apply more as the skin absorbs it and cover with gauze and a bandage.

Bach's Rescue Remedy
I carry this with me permanently and consider myself well equipped for any emergency with a bottle in my pocket. This deals with the emotional effects of shock which if not helped immediately can reverberate through the system for years, causing an insidious build-up of all sorts of psychological and physiological problems. When coupled with skullcap it is one of the best remedies for short-term stress. (One size 'O' capsule of the skullcap should be taken hourly as long as the acute crisis lasts.)

The rescue remedy should be diluted, 4 drops in 2 fl oz (60 ml) pure spring water to which a little brandy has been added as a preservative. Take 4 drops in 1 teaspoon water and hold it on the tongue for thirty seconds before swallowing. Repeat this at least four and up to six times daily. If the patient is unconscious, rub it into the lips or on the wrists. Rescue remedy is available from some health food shops or by post (see Appendix).

Blackberry bark, golden-seal and chaparral
For dysentery take an enema of thinned yoghurt if at all possible and every half hour take the size 'O' capsule of 2 parts blackberry bark mixed with 1 part golden-seal and 1 part chaparral.

Black peppercorns
Mix seven crushed peppercorns in a teaspoon of honey and chew slowly and thoroughly to relieve sore throats.

To accelerate the healing process of a fever chew sixteen black peppercorns followed by a drink of iced water. Take an Epsom salt bath and go to bed early wrapped up well in order to sweat it out.

Catnip and fennel tincture
To relieve flatulence, stomach cramps and colic as well as travel sickness take 1 teaspoon in a little water as often as needed.

Cayenne powder and cayenne tincture
For shock take 1 teaspoon of the powder in hot water. In the event of a heart attack take 3 teaspoons of the powder in a cup of water drunk immediately and all at once. Then take 10 drops of the tincture in hot water every quarter of an hour until normal colour returns and of course get medical help as quickly as possible.

To stop haemorrhaging internally or externally apply the powder directly to the wound; or mix it with water and use it as a douche or ingest the liquid orally. It is rich in vitamin A and so acts as an excellent disinfectant. For a nose-bleed sniff it. As a vaginal douche mix 1 oz (3 og) to 1 pint (600 ml) of warm water and administer it lukewarm and unstrained.

For toothaches, swelling or inflammation, rub on the tincture directly. For arthritis rub the tincture on the inflamed area and wrap round with a piece of red flannel (other colours really don't seem to be as effective!).

As a poultice mixed with equal parts of plantain, the powder is remarkably good for drawing out splinters.

Chickweed ointment
Apply externally to eczema or for genital itching. Alternatively apply marigold cream.

Cramp bark
For menstrual and muscle cramps take two size 'O' capsules of cramp bark as needed, but not more than eight daily.

Echinacea
Apply the tincture directly to snake or insect bites, and take 1 teaspoon in a little water every two hours.

Eucalyptus
For bronchitic chests dissolve 10 drops of the essential oil into 1 teaspoon of alcohol and add 5 drops of lobelia. Rub this liniment into the affected area.

Eyebright
For sore, red eyes wash out each eye with a fresh mixture of 2 drops of the tincture in an eyebath. Also, take 10 drops internally in a little water three times daily.

Fenugreek
To eliminate excess mucus and relieve congestion, make a decoction of 1 oz (30 g) of the crushed seeds with seven crushed peppercorns to 1 pint (600 ml) water. A decoction taken alone will relieve gout and hypoglycaemic symptoms.

Garlic
Apply a few drops of the oil in the ear to relieve earache. Take 1 tablespoon of the syrup to relieve a cough.

Ginger
To relieve travel sickness take a wineglassful of ginger tea made with the fresh root and sweetened with honey. Alternatively take

1 size 'O' capsule as often as needed. Also try 3 drops of essential oil of marjoram in a little honey water – particularly effective for seasickness.

Golden-seal tincture
Apply directly to herpes simplex, and if you can bear it chew a clove of garlic.

Juniper berries
In an emergency to induce urination chew the berries or drink a cup of the decoction. I once used this in such an emergency for someone who refused to urinate because the herpes sores on her genitals were so painful.

Lobelia
Mix this in apple cider vinegar as an emetic to get rid of inadvertently swallowed medicines. In the event of a severe asthmatic attack, give 1 teaspoon cayenne tincture and warm water followed by 1 teaspoon lobelia tincture. Repeat this lobelia dose two more times at fifteen-minute intervals. Wait for the patient to vomit to purge the bronchials of mucus. Then offer a cup of peppermint tea to soothe the stomach. Rub on the tincture externally to relieve muscular spasms.

Lower bowel tonic
To relieve constipation (see page 67).

Plantain
For stomach acidity take 1 teaspoon of the tincture in water as needed – or chew a small piece of calamus root.

Rosemary
Equal parts of tincture of rosemary and cayenne – 30 drops in water are needed to relieve headache. Alternatively massage 1 drop of lavender oil into each temple.

Thyme
As an external antiseptic use the tea freely to bathe the infected area. For bronchitis and laryngitis drink a wineglassful of the tea sweetened with plenty of honey and do not exceed 1 pint (600 ml) a day.

7

Menstruation

It seems that the average age of menarche (first menstruation) has been progressively declining over the last 100 years at the rate of one year in every generation. The oldest reliable records on menarche are Norwegian and date back to the 1850s when the average age for the first period was 17. By 1950 it had fallen to 13½. This may be because of better diet and healthier living conditions but it is also the result of our escalating ingestion of hormones hidden in various foods. In the Philippines little girls drinking from a stream where hormone-injected chickens were killed and washed were growing breasts and beginning periods at the age of 5. Biologists say that the age of puberty and menarche have reached their minimum genetic potential. I am not so sure. And the thing that saddens me is that we do not afford the menarche the celebration it deserves. There is nothing comparable to it in male physiology or as a rite of passage – it is not just a passing into womanhood but a declaration of the capacity to be a lover. Women seem to regard their bleeding angrily, evasively or with distaste; some try to make it anonymous, and you have only to look at the language surrounding menstruation to appreciate this – 'the curse', 'aunty', 'it', 'the time of the month', 'the usual', 'having a period', 'coming on'.

The blood itself is a harmless mixture that contains thirty times as much lime as regular blood and so lacks the chemical requirements for clotting. But the whole phenomenon is steeped in myth and the sight of a woman menstruating has revolted men, striking them with unwarranted terror so that they have devised rigid prohibitions for menstruating women that have kept them from love-making, from seeing the sun or touching the earth. It seems that the myth that says that menstrual blood is unclean is still very much alive and many men are still aghast at the thought of getting it on their penis or any other part of them. And the sadness is that many women have concurred in this and, unconvinced of the naturalness of their monthly bleeding, go to great lengths to hide it and obscure its odour. I still know people who will not wash their hair during menstruation, believing that it will increase the flow and make colds more likely.

The advertising industry wants us to believe that bleeding should be sanitized, whitened, neat, sweet and discreet. I absolutely disapprove of internal sanitary 'protection' (I use the word advisedly) for several reasons. I have observed in my own clinic that it heightens a woman's susceptibility to thrush and other vaginal problems. It is not unheard of to leave the last one behind – silly though that may sound. There have also been instances of toxic shock as the result of inserting tampons over broken skin. Some of my patients tell me that they feel tampons soak up all their bodily fluids, not just blood, leaving them feeling uncomfortably dried out after menstruation.

Having therefore come down on the side of sanitary towels, I should at the same time caution you always to wipe your bottom front to back. If you don't do so, and you wear a sanitary towel during menstruation, you are in danger of inadvertently spreading unwanted bacteria from the anus to the vagina, because the sanitary towel tends to move a little as the body moves. Wiping from front to back is always a good idea but especially when bacteria are more easily moved forward by a sanitary towel.

It is during menstruation that a bidet really comes into its own, making it much easier to wash the vulva, vagina and anus. There is no need to use soap while using a bidet. The free flow of warm water is perfectly adequate for cleansing. Pat, do not rub, afterwards with a towel. Rubbing may only result in unwanted irritation.

During a normal period you will lose only about 4 tablespoons of actual blood (that is 2 fl oz or 60 ml) over four or five days. The remaining 3–4 fl oz (90–120 ml) is made up of water, mucus and other fluids married with fragments of decomposing tissue shed from the interior of the uterus and several million epithelial cells that flake off the lining of the vagina. You will need a little extra iron during menstruation as you lose 15–30 mg so if you feel you are not ingesting enough iron-rich food take the formula on page 177.

Menstrual Pain

Menstruation should not be painful. My only painful periods were when, in my ignorance, I was fitted with a copper IUD, and once after a three-week grape fast, when I took the unusual period to be part of the deep cleansing process.

If cramping is severe it is because the uterus is heavily burdened with a highly toxic discharge and because calcium levels have dropped too low, causing muscle spasm and debility. The level of calcium in the bloodstream drops a week beforehand and even more so at the onset of menstruation, so take the calcium formula on page 175 for the week before menstruation is due, and stick to warm foods only. Take warm sitz-baths or saunas to relax the uterus and ease the flow. Do not let your breathing become cramped and shallow. If blood is bright red it is indicative of poor assimilation of sugars and carbohydrates. If it is dark red, stringy or smelly, it shows that the body is overburdened with putrefying protein and you should cut down on all meat, eggs and dairy products. The ideal colour of healthy menstrual blood is reddish brown.

Pain immediately before menstruation suggest that the position of the womb is abnormal. This is often seen in very thin women in whom the internal fat and ligament upon which the uterus is suspended has lost its tone. Let me clarify the conception of a normal position for a uterus. A uterus which is tipped towards the spine is called 'retroverted'. If it tips towards the pelvic bone it is called 'antiverted'. If it bends over itself it is called 'retroflexed' or 'antiflexed'. There seems to be a gynaecological obsession with uterine positioning, but a tipped uterus is not a 'condition' a woman need to worry about. Most women's uteri point in different directions at different times in their lives, but there are very few women who have a uterus tipped to such a degree that it causes pain or makes any difference in their ability to become pregnant.

If the uterus truly is out of position, slant-board exercises (see Chapter 3) will help this, as will the exercises mentioned on page 171. If pain is before menstruation but not just before, this suggests that the ovaries may be unhealthy, in which case hot sitz-baths should be taken on alternate nights the week before menstruation is due. Eliminate all processed and refined foods and emphasize raw and sprouted seeds, nuts, raw organically grown fruit and vegetables, plenty of raw juices and supplementations of kelp, lecithin and cold-pressed vegetable oils used uncooked as salad dressings. The formula on page 152 will also help, as will raspberry and figwort poultices placed over the abdomen. If pain is felt during the menstrual flow it means your womb is inflamed and crying out for help and at this juncture you will need the help of a medical herbalist.

Unhappily I have met too many women who come into my clinic telling me about cysts 'the size of an orange' who have suffered in silence for years rather than get help. Most of them are beyond middle age and I suspect they have been brought up with the old-fashioned idea that a little pain with menstruation is natural and all part of a woman's lot. This is rubbish – menstruation should be comfortable and easy throughout life. If it is not, there is almost certainly something wrong, so do not ignore it – put it at the top of your list of urgent priorities.

HERBAL FORMULAE FOR MENSTRUAL PAIN

For painful cramping menstruation

If menstruation comes with severe cramping pain, sip cups of the following tea taken as hot as possible sitting quietly and comfortably. Drink it between meals or better still while fasting.

> 2 parts mugwort
> 2 parts cramp-bark
> 1 part pasque-flower
> 1 part peppermint
> 1 part wild yam

Take this as often as needed while the cramping lasts. In-between use warm hand and foot baths made with equal parts of elderflowers, marigold, spearmint and sage, and during the rest of the month use these twice daily, morning and evening.

An alternative which will, given time, regulate your menstural cycle and ease discomfort is:

Dr Christopher's periodic formula

> 2 parts cramp-bark
> 2 parts squaw vine

1 part true unicorn root
1 part beth root
1 part blue cohosh
1 part pennyroyal
1 part cascara sagrada
1 part allspice

Take 2–3 size 'O' capsules of the finely powdered herbs with each meal throughout the month. As the effect is cumulative you will find that you need less and less each month while the body learns to regulate itself.

EXERCISES FOR MENSTRUAL PAIN

It is very tempting to curl up in bed hugging a hot-water bottle and feeling sorry for yourself. Don't. Force yourself to do the following exercises even though it may be the last thing in the world you actually feel like doing.

1. Lie on your back at right angles to the wall with your buttocks as near to the wall as possible. Prop your feet up against the wall, ensuring that the soles are flat and the knees a little bent. Stay there for five minutes.
2. Now move away from the wall and bring one leg up as close to your chin as you can get it. Leave the other on the floor. Hold the lifted leg up with your arms to take the strain and now hold that position for two minutes. Then swap round using the other leg.
3. Get up so that you are resting on your knees and elbows, stretching your head and arms out so that your elbows are on the ground in front of you with your head between your arms. (This is also helpful for those who have pain immediately after intercourse just before a period.)
4. Regular walking, running, skipping, swimming or horse-riding also helps. Women who are not very physically active get more problems than active ones both with menstrual pain and pregnancy and delivery.

Reflexology for the Lower Back and Female Organs

Find the reflexology pressure point for the lower back, which is at the base of the arch on both feet near the heel. Sit comfortably in a

Pressure Points for Female Organs

Inside view of foot

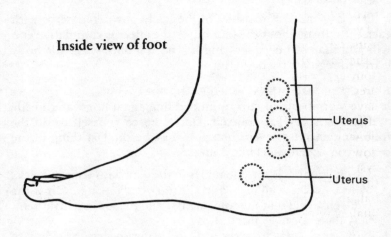

Uterus

Uterus

Outside view of foot

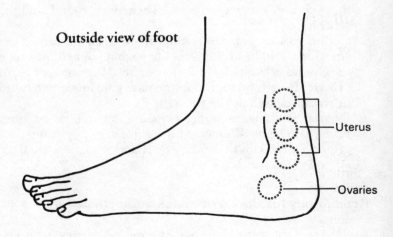

Uterus

Ovaries

chair. Put your foot in your lap so that you can get at the sole. Now press on the lower-back reflexology point with your thumbs. (Make sure your thumbnails are nice and short of course.) This will ease lower-back pain.

The reflexology pressure points for the genitals and female organs are also around the ankle. Press on the inside of your foot on a spot about halfway between your ankle bone and the bottom of your heel for affecting the uterus. Press on a similar spot on the outside of your foot for affecting the ovaries. Squeeze and pinch either side of your Achilles tendon about 3 in (7.5 cm) up from your heel — another point for affecting the uterus. In each case press firmly. If it feels tender or hurts, ease up but do not stop. I have taught patients to use this technique with remarkably good effect. If menstruation is usually very heavy, these areas should be worked on throughout the month but *not* during the actual flow as this will make the flow even heavier. Fibroid tumours and cysts also respond well to reflexology, but as the pituitary and thyroid reflexes need to be worked on to restore glandular balance I would suggest that in this instance you consult a qualified reflexologist.

Other Menstrual Problems

ADJUSTING THE FLOW

For excessively heavy menstruation

> 2 parts shepherd's purse
> 1 part lovage
> 1 part geranium root
> ½ part ginger

Make a tincture and take 1 teaspoon three times daily with meals. Concentrate on iron-rich foods (see page 177), especially a little watercress juice expressed into and mixed with beetroot juice. If the excessive flow carries on over several menstruations consult a gynaecologist to ensure that it is not indicative of something more serious.

To help the flow during menstruation

Equal parts of:

 yellow dock
 burdock
 red clover
 nettles
 parsley
 cinnamon

Drink half a cup of the infusion every two hours for the duration of your period.

If you want to get rid of a period quickly there is also a method of period extraction available in some well-woman clinics where a special tube, called a cannula, attached to a suction device, is inserted into the uterus when the period starts and the menstrual fluid is sucked out in five minutes. It is a convenient technique but my reservations are that it must be practised in absolutely sterile conditions by experts on women who have never had pelvic inflammatory disease, and as yet the possible long-term effects on the uterus are unknown. Besides which we do not yet know what this does to the delicate co-operation between the hypothalamus and the pituitary gland. The hypothalamus responds to the low levels of oestrogen by directing the pituitary to release FSH (female sex hormone) so that the proliferative phase can begin anew. Accelerate the process artificially and we could be in trouble in the long run. So consider this only in an emergency and accept that bleeding is part of being sexual.

The flow of blood can actually be a pleasurable experience. I find that taking a sauna or Turkish bath helps, as does taking a long hot soak in a bath with a teaspoon of motherwort oil added and a few drops of rose oil for its soothing fragrance. Fasting on the first day, drinking only hot herbal teas, helps and makes you feel lighter and more aware and in touch with yourself.

METRORRHAGIA

This is spotting between periods. Take hand or foot baths of equal parts of:

 marshmallow
 blackberry leaves

sage
chasteberries
hawthorn
garlic

Make sure that you have plenty of iron and calcium in your diet. The formula recommended to help the flow during menstruation is also helpful. If the condition persists in spite of an exemplary diet and exercise programme and the faithful ingestion of these two formulae for more than a few months, seek the advice of a medical herbalist.

AMENORRHOEA

This is when you do not menstruate at all. Periods may fail to appear for all sorts of reasons other than pregnancy – stress or physical illness, for example. In particular, it is common for the periods that follow the menarche to be irregular and the bleeding short or lengthy. Ovulation is inevitably a bit hit-or-miss during these irregular cycles, which can go on for up to six years until the body settles down to its own hormonal cycle (generally between 24 and 34 days, 28 days being average). Uterine tonics like rue, southernwood, false unicorn or blue cohosh can help the body to attain its natural cycle more speedily.

These will help in adulthood too but you may need something stronger to bring on menstruation. A cup of an infusion of equal parts of pennyroyal, parsley and tansy drunk three times daily on an empty stomach between meals is very effective. But as some of these herbs are abortifacients be sure that you are not pregnant before taking them.

If the problem is more deeply entrenched, try the following formula on a regular basis for six months:

2 parts tansy
2 parts catnip
1 part pennyroyal
1 part rosemary
1 part chasteberry
½ part cinnamon

Take two size 'O' capsules of the finely powdered herbs with each meal with a wineglassful of a tea made with raspberry and squaw vine mixed in equal parts. Adjust the diet to include plenty of hormone-rich foods like banana, wholegrains, sprouted seeds, bee pollen, royal jelly and natural liquorice.

ENDOMETRIOSIS

The blanket that lines the uterus in which the fertilized egg is planted is called the endometrium. Inadequate hygiene before, during or after love-making (for example a dirty finger, or one that has been previously inserted into the anus and not washed, inserted into the vagina), childbirth, abortion, uterine curettage, and carelessly inserted forceps are all means of introducing harmful bacteria into the endometrium. Poor diet and lifestyle, a wrongly positioned womb, retained placenta, lead poisoning and blood disorders also leave the uterus vulnerable to infection. Endometriosis begins when small nests of cells 'stray' into the pelvis, ovaries, fallopian tubes and bladder, forming tiny cysts. They bleed with the rest of the endometrium with each menstruation but are not evidenced until the cysts are stretched and swollen, which may take ten or fifteen years. Endometriosis afflicts 5–10 per cent of women between the ages of twenty-five and forty-five, and symptoms include chronic lower abdominal pain, dysmenorrhoea, pain after love-making and infertility.

The herbal approach is two-prolonged. First clear up the infection as speedily as possible, and second take herbs naturally rich in hormones. Echinacea and golden-seal are both excellent antiseptic herbs. Squaw vine, blessed thistle and liquorice are all rich in hormones. Use the following treatments together.

First douche every day with equal parts of golden-seal, echinacea and squaw vine, retaining the douche as long as possible (at least twenty minutes). Also take the following formulation:

3 parts echinacea
1 part golden-seal
1 part squaw vine
1 part blessed thistle
1 part parsley
1 part marshmallow
1 part cayenne
1 part liquorice

Take two size 'O' capsules of the finely powdered herbs with each meal. If the condition does not improve considerably in six months seek the advice of a professional medical herbalist.

It may sound strange, but the absence of ovulation and menstruation will affect a cure in many cases. This means that if you are a young woman intending to have a family at some point the solution may well be the simple one of getting pregnant. If the problem recurs, you could consider spacing children closer together rather than waiting. In other words, endometriosis can be alleviated by interrupting normal ovarian function, and it is for this reason that it often spontaneously improves once the menopause starts. Above all, remember that complete recovery may well be possible if the disease is diagnosed and treated early. So do not hesitate to seek the advice of a gynaecologist if in doubt. The blood-filled sacs, which can range from the size of a pinhead to that of a walnut and which are dark blue or purple, can easily be detected by fibre-optic examination or laparoscopy.

PREMENSTRUAL TENSION

This is becoming so widely recognized that they are even making television programmes about it, and some say it is the commonest cause of all marital break-down. Shoplifting apparently is thirty times more common premenstrually.

The symptoms fall into two categories, emotional and physical, but rest assured that the cause does not simply lie in your head. Many of the physical changes are the result of a shift in fluid balance in response to progesterone, which is produced in large quantities following ovulation. Common physical changes include swelling of the breasts, feet and hands, haemorrhoids, weight gain, migraines, backache, cramping, painful joints, pimply blotched skin and lank hair, asthma, hayfever, hoarseness and red eyes. Common emotional ones include food and alcohol cravings, depression, fatigue and irritability.

The intensity of the emotional shift varies from woman to woman and month to month, and much depends on how you feel about menstruating. Do you regard it as unclean, secret, embarrassing, or difficult, or as a special time to be acknowledged and honoured? Much depends on your attitude (which will be partly determined by your upbringing) and the degree of hormonal shifting in the critical days before a period.

Good diet is a prerequisite for wholistic help with premenstrual tension, as is plenty of rest, total abstention from alcohol at this time, talking about your feelings and keeping a premenstrual chart so that any untoward symptoms do not catch you or those you love – who get the brunt of your irritability – by surprise. Supplements taken throughout the month should include 1,000 IU vitamin E (as long as you do not suffer from hypertension or a rheumatic heart complaint), as well as 300 mg vitamin B_6, increasing to 500 mg the week before a period, 1 strong B-complex tablet and 6 capsules evening primrose oil daily. If water retention is a problem, drink copious amounts of dandelion tea or dandelion root coffee. The following formulation is a general one designed to help water retention, cramping, nervous tension and nutritional and metabolic strain on the body.

3 parts dandelion
2 parts horsetail
1 part motherwort
1 part wild yam
1 part pasque-flower
1 part scullcap
1 part lady's-slipper
1 part borage
1 part kelp
1 part cinnamon

Take one size 'O' capsule of the finely powdered herbs hourly with sips of sarsaparilla tea. Once the premenstrual tension has eased, reduce to three size 'O' capsules three times daily with meals throughout the month.

WATER RETENTION
If this is your only problem with menstruation, drink a tea made of equal parts of dandelion, cleavers, yarrow and bear-berry. Drink this copiously as long as the water retention lasts. You should also, of course, cut out salt and increase your potassium intake.

CHANGES IN BOWEL MOVEMENTS
Many women experience radical changes in bowel movements just before or while menstruation. I have observed this over the years with many of my patients. Part of the reason may be that

stress is hindering normal peristalsis of the colon, but some of it is the way hormones influence the body. Either way, ensure that your diet is full of fibre and that you drink plenty of liquid, and take the lower bowel tonic (see page 67) and nerve tonic (see pages 173 and 205) if you feel these are necessary, or the formula on page 163 if the problem is hormone-related. Ensure that your calcium intake is high. Take alternating hot and cold sitz-baths, splashing water liberally over the abdomen.

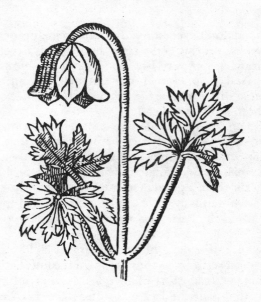

8

Conception

Many women don't even know they are pregnant for the first six to eight weeks, yet this is the time the foetus is developing very rapidly, drawing her very life-blood from her mother. So it is obviously vital to prepare for pregnancy way in advance of conception in order to give the best possible chance of optimum health to both mother and child.

A Canadian study revealed that nearly six times as many women on an inadequate diet before and during pregnancy had uncomfortable complications including nausea, anaemia, threatened miscarriage, toxaemia and varicose problems, compared with those on a good diet. It was particularly striking that although a woman may have *appeared* to be healthy on a poor diet, very often the baby was born in extremely poor physical condition.

We pass on our genetic blueprints to our children, and sadly they tend to get scruffier as they go down the line. So if you come from a family with a history of allergies, asthma or hay fever, it is more likely that your children will suffer from the same problem. If your child has to wear glasses or has a mouthful of fillings in spite of a reasonable diet, the chances are that you, your parents and even their parents have all been lacking in adequate nutrition, and the problem has been exacerbated generation by generation. It is possible to change this dismally predictable pattern by looking to your own state of health *well before* you attempt to conceive. Far better to prepare and prevent than repair and repent!

If you have a particular health problem and you are planning a family some time in the future, resolve to put all your energies *now* into eliminating or at least alleviating it. If you have or have had in the past, an unhealthy lifestyle – perhaps involving a junk-food diet, smoking, heavy drinking, drugs, obesity or lack of exercise – allow yourself at least a year to prepare for a really healthy conception.

You can go a step further and contribute to the health of future generations by bringing up your own children with a clear understanding of the philosophy behind your diet and life-style. This is probably the greatest and most durable gift you can pass on to your children. Be persistent and make it fun, so that good health and all that its maintenance entails become second nature to your children and not just one of 'Mum's little quirks'.

My god-daughter will willingly eat even the bitterest of herbal tablets because she has never been given any allopathic medication and has consumed very little sugar. She actually asks for her favourite herbal teas. Remember too that allopathic drugs can be stored in the body for years, usually settling in a long-suffering liver, and can be passed on to the foetus via the placenta or in breast milk, so use natural remedies for all your ailments as far as you possibly can.

Pre-conception Cleansing

An excellent way to clean up the body prior to conception is to go on a grape fast for three to four weeks, eating 4–6 lb (2–3 kg) well-washed grapes daily. (Basil Shackleton's book *The Grape Cure* is particularly helpful here: see Bibliography.) After the period of the fast, gradually return to a normal diet as described in Chapter 1, taking the same amount of time to do so as you did fasting, and if you are not a vegetarian stick to chemical-free chicken and fresh fish by way of flesh products.

MEN NEED CLEANSING TOO
Potential fathers are not let off the hook. Dr Bayer, a German obstetrician, has stated that he'd never known a mentally handicapped child to be born provided the father took vitamin E on a regular basis for many months prior to conception. (The dosage depended on the history of diseases such as rheumatic fever and hypertension.)

In the Arab world it is customary to feed stallions on wild mint in order to increase their potency. So perhaps plenty of peppermint tea might be worth a try. The Arabs also recommend as generally strengthening a drink made of the powdered root of the wild orchid (*Orchis mascula*) sweetened with honey and served well spiced. This 'salep' was quite popular in this country before the proliferation of coffee houses and I have often encountered it in Turkey. Its taste is milky and pleasant and it is quite palatable.

Men should give up smoking and drinking, especially in the few months prior to attempting to conceive, and while the couple is attempting to conceive, in order to improve both the quality and quantity of sperm. It is advisable that they follow the same programme of diet and exercise as prescribed for their partner.

HEAVY METAL TOXICITY

Unhappily the air we breathe and many of the products we touch are full of toxic minerals which can cause both physical and mental problems. Lead, mercury, aluminium and cadmium are all toxic minerals which are increasingly threatening health in our industrial society. They have no use at all as far as the body is concerned, and prolonged exposure to them decreases vitality, shortens lifespan and generally aggravates disease.

Exhaust fumes are the main source of lead. Others are lead piping, the solder used on food cans, cigarette smoke and lead-based pottery and glazes. There is increasing evidence to suggest that raised body levels of lead lower IQ, decrease mental concentration, increase the chance of miscarriage, birth defects and still-births, can lead to criminal and delinquent behaviour in children, increase cancer rates and generally accelerate the ageing process.

Mercury is present in the fungicides used to protect grain, fish swimming in mercury-saturated seas, some fabric-softeners and floor waxes, mercury vapour lamps, some cosmetics and adhesives, and of course dental amalgams. Mercury, like lead, will cross the placental barrier during pregnancy, so that mothers exposed to it, though they may show no signs of mercury poisoning themselves, can produce babies which are grossly mentally and physically deformed. In the United States alone, about 450 tons of mercury a year are used in fungicides and insecticides. For every ton of chlorine produced, approximately 8 oz (250 g) mercury is released into the atmosphere – making the staggering quantity of over a million pounds a year in the USA. Amalgam fillings use approximately 50 per cent mercury, and present estimates show that (again, in the USA) about 100 tons mercury are used in dentistry every year and this amount is on the increase. Mercury breaks down in the fillings and is gradually absorbed into the body, causing many ailments, both minor and serious, which have only recently been attributed to mercury poisoning. Problems such as blurred vision, headaches, dizziness, depression and irritability can all be the result of mercury poisoning. Some brain tumours can be caused by mercury poisoning. If you are interested in the subject it is well worth reading *The Toxic Time Bomb* by Sam Ziff (see Bibliography).

Aluminium, in the form of aluminium kitchen-wear, aluminium foil, aluminated salts (this includes most table salt), baking powder, antacids, toothpaste, cigarette filters, buffered aspirin, cosmetics, hot-water heaters with aluminium heating elements, processed cheese, cosmetics and pharmaceuticals, is all around us. Symptoms of toxicity usually begin with persistent indigestion and lead on to gastrointestinal upsets, rickets (by interfering with phosphate absorption), cirrhosis, cystic fibrosis and senility. Aluminium reacts vigorously with alkaline saliva, so that by the time food cooked in aluminium saucepans reaches your stomach, gas is being produced in just the same way as baking powder acts on a rising cake. To some extent the hydrochloric acid in the stomach keeps this under control, but the situation is less happy in the duodenum. So never cook or bake in aluminium. Use iron, earthenware, china, glass, stainless steel or enamel-lined saucepans. Aluminium from aluminium saucepans goes on reacting and producing painful gas all the way through the colon, upsetting the delicate pH of the whole digestive tract, flooding the bloodstream and burdening the body's organs. Aluminium accumulates in the body, so the overall effect gets worse with age. Fortunately, it can be sped out of the body by eating foods high in pectin, particularly bananas, apples, lemons, lemon rind and sunflower seeds.

Smokers have much higher levels of cadmium in their livers than non-smokers, and it is also found in tap-water from galvanized or plastic water-pipes, tin cans, instant coffee, many processed meats, cola drinks, and refined cereals (which have a low zinc to cadmium ratio). Some scientists believe that cadmium is an even greater threat to health than either lead or mercury. Cadmium poisoning can result in hypertension, emphysema, arteriosclerosis, cerebral haemorrhage, kidney and liver damage, cystic fibrosis, cirrhosis and eventually a painful softening of the bones.

It is very hard to hustle cadmium (unlike lead and mercury) out of the body quickly, but cadmium antagonists are calcium, iron, protein, vitamin D and zinc. So protection against toxicity would seem to be provided by a diet of rich unprocessed foods and a reasonable degree of sunshine in as unpolluted an atmosphere as possible.

Once you have ensured that all six eliminative channels are functioning properly (see Chapter 3), it is excellent preventive medicine to embark on a heavy-metal cleanse as almost all of us have too much lead, mercury, aluminium and cadmium in the system. *Do not* undertake a heavy-metal cleanse unless the eliminative channels are working well, otherwise you will experience weakness, dizziness, headaches and nausea. This is an extremely deep level of cleansing and is best undertaken in three-week periods, so you do three weeks on and three weeks off, over a period of three to four months.

Heavy-metal detoxification programme

1. Two level teaspoons of kelp powder or, two sheets of dulse, nori, seaweed or laver, daily.

2. One cup of homemade apple sauce. (Cook the apple with a squeeze of lemon juice and plenty of grated lemon rind in a tightly covered saucepan over a low heat.) During digestion the apple pectin is transformed into galacturic acid, which combines with the toxic metals to form an insoluble metallic salt, which is then excreted. Perhaps surprisingly, homemade apple sauce is a better-utilized source of pectin, as far as the body is concerned, than fresh apple.

3. Calcium is mopped up in advance of lead in the digestive tract, so high levels will act as a buffer against lead absorption. Don't think that you should be consuming lots of dairy products in order to boost calcium levels. Besides being mucus-forming, they actually increase lead absorption. There are other natural sources of calcium, such as oatmeal,

millet, bone-meal, alfalfa, sesame seeds, tahini, parsley, wheatgerm and camomile. Take 800 mg daily.

4. Vitamin E is known to be a protective agent in metal toxicity, so ensure that you get 800–1,000 IU daily (unless you have a history of rheumatic heart fever or hypertension).

5. Vitamin C is an extremely powerful anti-toxin, so take a minimum of 4–5 gm daily.

6. Vitamin A helps to activate the enzymes that will detoxify poisonous metals, so eat plenty of the gold-, orange- and red-coloured plants. If taking a supplement, combine vitamins A and D – 25,000 IU vitamin A with an appropriate balancing amount of D (2,500 IU). Take this for only two out of the three weeks you are doing the heavy-metal detoxification, so that your liver does not get overburdened with it (it will store what it doesn't immediately need).

7. Try and eat a couple of cloves of raw garlic daily or, if this is too antisocial, take six garlic perles daily with meals. Like the seaweeds, garlic is rich in the sulphur-containing amino-acids. If you can't bring yourself to take the garlic, use onions instead but you will need more, about two daily, which are best taken in onion soup. Alternatively, use half a cup of cooked kidney beans or broadbeans daily which will carry out the same task.

8. Take daily Epsom salt baths (see Chapter 6) to encourage elimination through the skin.

9. As the kidneys get particularly heavily burdened by the toxic metals pouring out of the system, drink three wineglassfuls of parsley tea daily, and ensure that your liquid intake is kept high.

10. Take the following formula:

3 parts gipsy-weed
3 parts yellow dock
1 part chaparral
1 part plantain
1 part lobelia

Take three size 'O' capsules of the finely powdered herbs morning and evening.

Try to get aluminium out of your life; and, if you possibly can, cut down your exposure to lead by living away from a town or city centre or main road. Certainly children should not live within 200 yd (180 m) of a motorway. Be careful where you buy your vegetables. Those grown in large cities are liable to be heavily polluted.

RADIATION POISONING

When news of the Chernobyl nuclear accident reached Britain the phone lines of organizations like the Friends of the Earth and the Campaign for Nuclear Disarmament were jammed by worried people wanting to know whether to drink milk, whether their water was safe, whether they could eat vegetables or allow their children to play outside. The bland reassurance of an indifferent government resulted not so much in panic as in an understandable demand for reliable, practical advice. On a recent BBC 'Panorama' programme it was revealed that the limits set by the government for exposure to radiation may be more than ten times too high. It seems that safety limits are based on estimates of acceptable risks, and a one in 100,000 risk of cancer is seen to be acceptable – that is, approximately 600 extra deaths a year in this country from cancer. The radiation exposure limits are calculated on the basis of figures for *deaths* from cancer rather than those suffering from cancer. This further increases their inaccuracy. It is only now being understood that some people are much more sensitive to radiation than others.

Quite apart from this, the official safety limits for exposure do not reflect the scientific estimates of risk anyway. When legislation for this country was being drawn up last year, the International Commission for Radiological Protection recommended that a limit of 1 millisievert (unit of radiation) per year be set for public exposure to radiation. Instead a limit of 5 millisievert was adopted.

People around Sellafield are exposed to levels of radiation of about 2–3 millisieverts, so accepting a limit of just 1 would clearly cause problems for the government.

Radiation is known to cause cancer, and the rates of leukaemia among children living near Sellafield are nine times higher than the national average. Radiation is known to cause cancers of the breast and thyroid, of the lung, stomach, liver, large intestine, bone, oesophagus, small intestine, urinary system, pancreas, rectum and lymphatic tissues in roughly that order of frequency.

The genetic damage caused by radiation may result in death, disease and disability to children as yet unborn for many generations to come. Rough calculations by British experts on the worldwide effect of the Chernobyl disaster, using scanty evidence and optimistic assumptions, suggest that, between 10 and 100 people will die from the first three waves, and there will be 1,000–10,000 extra cancers over the next forty years.

It is estimated that background radiation causes 1–2 per cent of cancers, i.e. 2,000 a year in the UK. If the level of background radiation is higher, proportionately more cancers will result. In the week of the Chernobyl cloud, the increase above the normal annual dose for natural radiation averaged over people of all ages was 15 per cent in the north and 1 per cent in the south of the country. Averaged over all ages and areas the increase was 4 per cent.

Radiation damages by smashing molecules. Some of these broken fragments, known as free radicals, are highly reactive and can disrupt normal cell metabolism.

Help against radiation

The best way to counter any damage is to take large quantities of vitamin C which acts as a free-range scavenger. Take a dose that stops just short of inducing diarrhoea. (My dose tends to be 9 g but this varies from person to person.) Vitamin C with bioflavonoids is a helpful long-term antidote to damage from all kinds of pollution.

Buckwheat is the only herb I know of which will help with radiation damage. Take three size 'O' capsules of the dried finely powdered herb three times daily.

Contraception

If couples are using oral contraception, I advise them to switch to another method for at least six months before trying to conceive a baby. The Pill can cause many unpleasant side-effects in some women, including migraine, oedema, depression, weight gain, extreme mood changes, circulation problems and nausea, and recently it has been linked to both cancer of the cervix and cancer of the breast. There is also a school of thought which suggests that children born to a woman who has been taking the Pill for many years could develop sexual problems as they grow up. It takes some months for the Pill to be totally removed from the body and for a normal menstrual cycle to re-establish itself. Use the sheath, a diaphragm or the 'temperature' method. The latter is only advisable if you have a full understanding of it. Do not use a copper IUD as it depletes zinc levels in the body. While coming off the Pill, take one of the pre-conception formulae given below.

PRE-CONCEPTION HERBAL FORMULAE
Any of the following herbs will help to tone and balance the body gynaecologically: red raspberry, squaw vine, tansy (which should not be taken during pregnancy), pennyroyal (which should not be taken during pregnancy), blessed thistle (which acts as an excellent tonic when drunk cold), false unicorn (which is excellent for both male and female reproductive organs), cramp-bark, blue cohosh, true unicorn root.

Female tonic

1 part true unicorn root
1 part squaw vine

Make a standard infusion and take half a cup 3–6 times daily. Or:

4 parts squaw vine
1 part true unicorn
1 part cramp-bark
1 part wild yam

Make a decoction and take 2–3 tablespoons three times daily.

Dr Christopher's female reproductive formula
This is designed to tone, strengthen and regulate the gynaecological organs, rebuilding, harmonizing and healing the reproductive system. It should not be used in isolation but needs to be coupled with a herbal programme aimed at cleansing any weak eliminative channels. For women with menstrual problems it should be used in conjunction with the formula on page 163.

3 parts golden-seal
1 part blessed thistle

1 part cayenne
1 part cramp-bark
1 part false unicorn
1 part ginger
1 part red raspberry
1 part squaw vine
1 part uva-ursi

Drink one cup of the tea morning and evening.

Hormone herbal combination

This is helpful for correcting hormone balance and then maintaining the proper balance in both women and men.
Equal parts of:

black cohosh
sarsaparilla
ginseng
blessed thistle
liquorice
false unicorn
wild yam
squaw vine
garlic

Take three size 'O' capsules of the finely powdered herbs morning and evening. For women, ensure that the ginseng is Siberian. For men, it should be Asiatic.

Prostate formula

The following formula combined with the bowel and lymph cleansing programme (see Chapter 3) will strengthen the male prostate gland.
Equal parts of:

hydrangea root
gravel root
marshmallow root
parsley
ginger
cayenne
buchu

golden-seal
echinacea
yellow dock root
mullein
burdock

Take three size 'O' capsules of the finely powdered herbs morning and evening for eight weeks with a cup of pumpkin-seed tea. Pumpkin seeds are rich in a male androgen hormone which will also cleanse the prostate gland. Make up the tea as a decoction, remembering to crush the seeds well first.

Shaping Up Internally and Externally

Limp, lazy parents tend to produce children in much the same mould, so work on your physical fitness with an exercise programme that has been individually designed for you. It should involve forms of exercise that you enjoy, otherwise you won't stick to it. Women should concentrate on exercises to strengthen the muscles of the pelvic floor (see page 171). Ensure that you are eliminating and assimilating effectively (see Chapters 1–3).

If you are very overweight or underweight (10 lb/4.5 kg either way doesn't matter much) try to correct the problem before conception by first finding out the reasons for it – whether they be glandular, psychological, emotional, metabolic or the result of hyperactivity.

UNDERWEIGHT?
Nearly 30 per cent of women in their twenties are underweight, and 35 per cent are underweight in their thirties. They may not have diagnosable anorexia nervosa but they are still in a state of less than optimum health.

If the insurance charts say that you are underweight, but you look great, feel terrific and have plenty of energy, you have got absolutely nothing to worry about. But if you get tired quickly, feel nervy and become ill easily, it's time you put on some weight. Develop a diet rich in whole grains and pulses, with reasonable amounts of cold-pressed oils and natural sweets like halva and nut and seed cereal bars. Go for quality not quantity – lentil soup with wholemeal bread and butter rather than cream cakes. Refined sweets and carbohydrates rob the appetite, displacing foods that have real value. Half a cup of nuts daily will help you put on nearly a pound (about 0.5 kg) a week. Half a large avocado is 185 calories – and that's without a dressing.

If you are nervy, learn to calm down, so that you digest your food properly. Don't feel that you shouldn't take exercise – it will help you put on weight in the right places. The following formula will help with digestion and ensure that nutrients are properly distributed through the bloodstream.

4 parts dandelion
1 part gentian
1 part wild yam
1 part fennel
1 part blessed thistle
1 part marigold
1 part ginger

Take two size 'O' capsules of the finely powdered herbs at the beginning of each meal with sips of unsweetened pineapple juice. Also ensure that your diet is rich in foods containing zinc. These include green leafy vegetables, brewer's yeast, all the seeds and, especially, liver.

OVERWEIGHT?

Attributing excess weight to over-eating is no more helpful than ascribing alcoholism to over-drinking. The main cause of over-eating is disordered appestat function (the appestat is the neural centre in the hypothalamus that controls appetite). The hypothalamus houses two food-consumption mechanisms, the hunger and the satiety centres. It is possible that impaired appestat function can be induced in the foetus by poor prenatal nutrition but even in this case it doesn't have to be a lifelong handicap.

Meals should be small and often to correct this (one large meal a day increases the cholesterol and phospholipid levels). Appestat function can also be disrupted by negative emotions – self-loathing, anxiety, fear, depression, jealousy – so it is extremely important to correct the underlying cause, approaching the whole problem of weight loss steadily and gently on a psychological level. Overweight people need a healthy sense of self-worth if they are to put things right.

On a more straightforward level, excess weight is indisputably the result of expending too little energy in relation to the amount of food you take in, so the simple answer is less food and more vigorous regular exercise. An additional benefit of exercise is that it can actually cut down the appetite.

Programme for weight loss

1. Avoid sugar in all its forms, natural or otherwise, including honey, maple syrup and black strap molasses.
2. Take 2 tablespoons cider vinegar in water before each meal.
3. Eat five or six small meals of unrefined food per day. Small meals minimize the conversion of food into fat and tend to keep hunger at bay.
4. On no account cut oil out of your diet completely. A small amount of natural oil encourages the combustion of food and gives a satisfied feeling after eating because it slows down the digestion of protein.
5. Avoid tea, coffee, alcohol and salt.
6. Get out and do something in the evenings which doesn't involve food. If your life pattern is anything like mine you don't have time to be tempted during the day because you are so busy but once you are relaxing at home it is easy to nibble.
7. Take 2 tablespoons lecithin daily.
8. Don't skip meals. If you do so, fat pours into the bloodstream at a level six times higher than normal which is burdensome for the heart.
9. Start an exercise programme and stay with it.
10. Skin-scrub twice daily.
11. Learn to love and value yourself and get the support of somebody both knowledgeable and sympathetic behind you – someone who doesn't have tunnel vision about the basic high protein-diet which seems to be the only way westerners think of losing weight.
12. Avoid those powders which, mixed with milk or water, are supposed to accelerate weight loss. They lack fibre and without fibre you are in danger of encouraging the formation of gall-stones.

Ensure that the bowel, kidneys and liver are working properly before going on a prolonged diet. Resort to blood-purifiers and kidney-cleansers in the final stages of a diet to help you over the final hump. In the meanwhile take the following formulation.

2 parts chickweed
1 part kelp
1 part black walnut leaves
1 part alfalfa
1 part horsetail
1 part plantain
1 part Irish moss
2 parts Turkey rhubarb
1 part ginger

Take two size 'O' capsules of the finely powdered herbs twenty minutes before each meal with a cup of dandelion tea or coffee. This formulation is designed to support the thyroid, to help to cleanse the colon, kidneys and liver, to boost the metabolic rate and to ensure a correct sodium–potassium ratio.

Spirulena, an algae farmed in Mexico, is very nutritious and helpful if you have strong hunger cravings but should never be used if your lymphatic system is poor. Take 2 teaspoons powdered spirulena stirred into juice before every meal.

Boy or Girl?

The sex of a baby is determined by the father's sex chromosome and the only foolproof way to plan the sex of a baby is by artificial insemination. The following methods will give you a slightly better than average chance of conceiving a baby of the sex you want and is based on the fact that sperm with Y sex chromosomes (which produce boys) are smaller, faster, lighter and stronger than sperm with X sex chromosomes (which produce girls). The former thrive in an alkaline environment, the latter in an acid environment. The likelihood of conceiving a boy is increased if you abstain from love-making until ovulation occurs. To neutralize the acidity of the vaginal secretions (if you want a boy), douche with a very weak solution of sodium bicarbonate just before love-making. If it is a girl you want make love frequently just before ovulation occurs (and, obviously, continue to make love as ovulation occurs) and douche with diluted apple cider vinegar.

Infertility

If you have been trying unsuccessfully to conceive for more than six months and you are under thirty, check (by using a temperature chart and detecting the change in your cervical mucus) that you are not consistently making love on infertile days of the month. Bear in mind that anxiety about being infertile can inhibit conception. Having a holiday is a good way of helping you to relax. A woman's natural fertility declines after the age of thirty, but if you have had a child or a previous pregnancy and are unable to conceive contact your doctor. It is unusual to experience difficulties in conceiving a second or third child. The good news is that although precise causes of infertility in a couple are often difficult to establish, at least 50 per cent of infertile patients can be helped medically.

With repeated ejaculations the number of sperm in the ejaculate declines. A high live-sperm count per ejaculate is known to be essential for conception to take place. So if your partner has ejaculated several times over the preceding few days, conception is less likely to occur on the day you ovulate because his semen will contain insufficient sperm. For this reason it is probably best to abstain from sexual intercourse for two or three days before ovulation is expected to occur.

On the other hand, it is not advisable to abstain for too long since sperm can live in the male reproductive system for only about ten days. Consequently the number of healthy sperm in the ejaculate is known to be reduced in men who have not ejaculated for more than a week.

If a woman stands up and walks around immediately after making love most of the seminal fluid will leak out of her vagina. To give as many sperm as possible a chance of beginning their journey to the fallopian tube into which the egg-cell will be or has been released it is a good idea to lie quietly on the bed for twenty minutes or more after making love with the buttocks raised slightly on a pillow and the knees bent upward. By using this position the semen will be encouraged to bathe the cervix.

I would strongly advise all infertile women to have an iridology test. This will help to establish which of the many possible causes of infertility are relevant to them. From my own experience I have found too many infertile women think only of their reproductive organs when the problem is more likely to be auto-intoxication. The following formula is good for cleansing all the organs contained in the pelvic and abdominal area, for purifying the blood, regulating periods, reducing swelling and soothing any vaginal irritation, relaxing the nervous system and killing any parasites. It is also rich in iron, potassium and vitamins B and C. Infertile women should take extra vitamin E up to 1,200 IU a day, provided their blood pressure is normal and there is no history of rheumatic fever.

Equal parts of:

red clover blossom
golden-seal
parsley
dandelion
blessed thistle
false unicorn
marshmallow
comfrey
lobelia
ginger

Infuse and drink three or four cups daily. Do not neglect a good overall body cleanse (see Chapter 3).

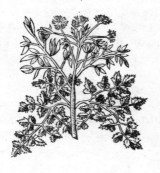

9

Pregnancy

Exercise

Pregnancy is not an illness, so don't treat yourself like Dresden china. Regular exercise will help to tone up the muscles and prepare the body for the exertion of childbirth. The sort of exercise you decide on very much depends on what you used to do before. Now is obviously not the time to start training for the Olympics if all you used to do is walk round to the local shop. The heart's workload increases by 40 per cent by the twenty-eight week so don't give it extra unnecessary work. If you were fairly active before, by all means keep it up, with the exception of water or snow skiing, parachuting, scuba-diving and horse-riding; and these are denied to you only because of the risk of injury. Any accident or fall during the early months of pregnancy could result in a miscarriage and when you're voluminous and your centre of gravity changes balancing can be difficult.

Swimming is wonderful and it is a blessed relief to be relieved of the weight of your bulk as you float in the water. Swimming is particularly helpful for relieving back pain. Obviously do not swim after a large meal, avoid very cold water as it may give you cramps, and don't try any high diving as the sudden change in your blood pressure could affect the baby's circulation.

Walking and dancing are great but don't get too acrobatic in the last few months (not that you are likely to feel like dominating a discothèque).

Yoga is good for harmonizing the body and the mind and for ensuring suppleness. Do remember to tell your yoga teacher that you are pregnant during the first few weeks when it will not show so that your teacher can ensure you are not practising unsuitable postures.

PELVIC-FLOOR EXERCISES

These are particularly important for pregnant women because learning to control the pubococcygeal muscle especially during the second stage of labour can help prevent tearing of the perineum. This PC muscle is a cone-shaped hammock suspended from the sides and back at the bottom of the pelvic bones, descending to the area between your legs. A weak PC muscle can cause menstrual problems, involuntary urination, a difficult pregnancy and delivery, infertility, painful intercourse, lack of sensation during love-making and difficulty in achieving orgasm, and can contribute to rectal, bladder and uterine prolapse. It is the only muscle in the body which is not exercised by gymnastics, daily living or any sport.

Testing the PC muscle

When you urinate spread your legs wide and try to stop the flow dead. Don't attempt this first thing in the morning or if you have recently drunk lots of liquid. If you can completely stop the flow several times consecutively you are in good shape. If not do the following exercise.

PC hold

It does not matter what position you adopt – sitting, standing or lying. Slowly contract the PC muscle (i.e. as though you were trying to stop urination) until you are squeezing it as forcefully as you can. Then hold the contraction. Count to ten slowly. Relax the muscle slowly. Breathe naturally throughout. No clenched teeth or thighs. Repeat ten times. If you can't hold each contraction for ten do what you can and build up slowly. Do not let the abdominal muscles assist the PC. You will know you are cheating if you lightly place your hand on the lower part of the abdomen during the exercise and feel it tightening. To avoid this, spread your legs.

I would advise every woman to exercise this muscle regularly from her teens on. Not only is a well-toned PC muscle beneficial during pregnancy but it is insurance against prolapses and incontinence later in life.

BAREFOOT WALKING

Walking barefoot on sand or grass will release the static

electricity in your body, so do it daily. Ensure that you dry your feet with a rough towel immediately afterwards to encourage your circulation.

Stress

As Juliette de Bairacli-Levy so beautifully put it, 'Pregnancy should be a daily song of triumph and thanksgiving in a woman's mind and heart.'

Stress is very common in pregnancy and burns up your nutrition faster than any other factor. Prolonged stress increases the chance of the baby suffering from neurological dysfunction, behavioural disturbances, developmental lags and generally poor health.

Hyperactive adrenal glands cause fatigue and exhaustion, so relaxation is if anything even more vital than exercise. The savasana (corpse pose) in yoga is very helpful, as is lying on the floor on cushions with your buttocks against the lower part of an armchair and your legs draped over the seat with bent knees. Two hours daily of complete relaxation is ideal and will help minimize labour pain.

STRESS SUPPLEMENTATION

The more carefully you buy and prepare your food, the less you will need in the way of supplements, but during times of stress it is not always possible to get all the vitamins you need through your diet alone. Supplement it with 25,000 IU vitamin A and 2,500 IU vitamin D; two strong sustained-release B-complex tablets, one after breakfast and one with lunch; 1,000 mg vitamin B_5; 6–9 g vitamin C sustained-release, divided into three doses taken with meals; and 1,000 IU vitamin E (provided your blood pressure is normal and there is no history of rheumatic fever).

Overworked adrenal glands can be supported with the following formulation.

Equal parts of:

mullein
borage
ginseng (preferably Siberian)

hawthorn
cayenne
gota kola
ginger
liquorice

Take ¼ level teaspoonful of the finely powdered herbs mixed with a little sugarless jam or juice three times daily. If you have any problems with high blood pressure, leave out the liquorice and the ginseng and substitute equal parts of motherwort and cinnamon. Take the supplementation suggested above together with this formulation only while under stress and for a few weeks afterwards.

Diet

I was astonished to read in a little book published by the British Medical Association that, 'Nothing very special is required for your diet in pregnancy. It is certainly unnecessary to add much to a diet that is normally well balanced.' A so-called well-balanced diet is extremely hard to achieve. Ninety-eight per cent of everything we eat passes through the hands (or more generally the machines) of food processors. The average Britain eats 4 lb (2 kg) of additives a year. Dr Williams has stated quite clearly that supermarket produce is likely to be deficient in vitamin B_6, magnesium, vitamin E, vitamin C, folic acid and trace minerals. A report in the *Sunday Times* (3 July 1983) investigating the four-year battle in Whitehall over Britain's calamitous dietary habits stated unequivocally, 'Anyone who eats the *average* British diet is in danger.'

A supine Department of Health aided and abetted by suppressions and evasions from complacent government ministers and compounded by the powerful lobbyists of the food manufacturing industry and the advertising industry will undoubtedly continue to perpetuate this situation. So forget all about 'average' and 'well balanced' and concentrate on superb.

Refer to Chapter 1 again and remember that, apart from the expectant mother's own nutritional requirements, by the time the foetus is six weeks old she will have stopped feeding off the amniotic sac and will be totally reliant on the mother for nourishment through the umbilical cord. It certainly is not necessary to 'eat for two' during pregnancy but you should aim for about 1,800 calories a day to avoid your baby being underweight at birth.

PROTEIN

The entire structure of your baby's body and brain will be largely made from the protein you eat, and your own need for protein includes that required for the formation of new tissue in the uterus and breasts. Ensure protein intake is at least 2½ oz (75 g) daily. Vegan mothers should make sure that they are getting enough combined foods (i.e. pulses married with grain, or grain married with legumes) to make a complete protein at any one sitting. I find that vegetarians and vegans with whom I work are generally more 'clued-up' about their protein requirements than meat-eaters, so this is usually not a problem.

Avoid gelatin (the least complete of all proteins) – it contains excessive glycine, which causes a protein imbalance that results in a slow seepage of essential amino-acids into the urine. Also, if you are prone to allergies try to take most of your protein from vegetarian sources that do not include high-protein foods like fish, eggs and dairy products. These (along with meat) are more allergenic than combination substitutes. By avoiding them you minimize the risk of passing your allergy on to your baby.

OILS AND FATS

Aim for 1–2 tablespoons of mixed vegetable oils daily and use them as part of a salad dressing (do not heat them). A teaspoon or so of unsalted butter is also permissible.

CALCIUM AND VITAMIN B₁₂

The need for calcium escalates rapidly during the last three months of pregnancy. A lack of it will cause leg and foot cramps, susceptibility to tooth decay (no doubt you have heard the quotation about a woman losing a tooth for every baby), headaches and sleeplessness. It may also lead to the baby having faulty bones and teeth.

It is difficult even in a healthy body to get calcium to pass into the bloodstream, and the problem is exacerbated by under-secretion of hydrochloric acid in the stomach. This generally comes about as the result of years of faulty diet. Lack of fat also means that calcium is more likely to be discarded in the faeces. Bear in mind too that vitamin B_{12} needs to be combined with calcium during absorption by the body to be of any real value.

There is a popular myth that vitamin B_{12} is only available in the animal and dairy products, and vegans are constantly lambasted about the possible deficiency of it in their diets. Actually 85 per cent of the vitamin B_{12} in meat is lost when it is cooked, and I do not know many people who indulge in steak tartare. Vitamin B_{12} is adequately manufactured by the bacteria in the intestines, provided the latter are not coated with mucus (which, of course, reduces the permeability of all vitamins), and provided putre-factive bacteria – from too much protein or sugar, or pollution or an enzyme deficiency – are not present.

Vitamin B_{12} is particularly abundant in four-day-old bean-sprouts (especially mung and alfalfa) and is present in sea plants, algae, rye, red clover, okra and sauerkraut as well as almonds, apples, asparagus, bananas, brewer's yeast, cantaloupe melons, carrots, celery, lemons, mushrooms, nuts, oranges, onions, parsley, peaches, cabbage, corn, comfrey, dates, grapes, grape-fruit, pineapple, rice polishings, soya-bean meal, spinach, tomatoes, watercress, watermelon, wheatgerm, wholewheat bread, and peas. Women with healthy intestines have a storage capacity sufficient to provide them with enough B_{12} for up to five years.

There is an equally popular myth that dairy products are the most effective form of calcium. They are *not*. An ounce (30 g) of hard cheese contains 230 mg calcium, compared to the 252 mg in 1 oz (30 g) watercress and 306 mg in 1 oz (30 g) kelp. Undoubted-ly plants are the best-assimilated form of calcium, and calcium needs vitamins A, C and D as well as phosphorus in order to function properly. Foods rich in calcium include oats, millet, sesame seeds, and most raw vegetables, especially turnip-tops and parsley. Pregnant women need 2,000 mg daily.

Calcium formula

6 parts horsetail
6 parts comfrey

3 parts nettles
2 parts kelp
1 part marshmallow root
1 part meadow-sweet
1 part lobelia

Take two size 'O' capsules of the finely powdered herbs with each meal throughout pregnancy. If you are feeling queasy with morning sickness mix the formula into honey and take it off the spoon.

IRON

The baby takes much of the mother's iron in the last two months of pregnancy and, like calcium, iron needs a healthy stomach excreting sufficient hydrochloric acid for its proper ingestion. A simple way to ensure this is to sip a teaspoon of cider vinegar in water half an hour before each meal.

Iron should *always* be taken in its natural form in foods and herbs and is most obvious in herbs with very dark green leaves. The inorganic iron salts used in the 'enrichment' of food are known to lead to chronic disability and fatal disease in some people. Natural sources of iron are far better assimilated in the body and in turn help with the assimilation of vitamins C and E. Natural iron has the added advantage of burning up accumulated poisonous waste, flushing it out of the body, and unlike synthetic iron it does *not* cause constipation. Coffee or products with caffeine in them, like chocolate, inhibit iron absorption.

Iron is richly present in rice polishings, kelp, wheatgerm, sunflower seeds, parsley and apricots, and to a lesser extent in purslane, the tops of beets and turnips, bilberry, blackberry, booklime, burdock, chicory, comfrey, cornflower, dandelion, yellow dock, gentian, groundsel, ground-ivy, hawthorn, hops, nettles, periwinkle, raspberry, restharrow, rose, salep, scabious, scullcap, strawberries, toadflax, vervain, watercress, wood-sage, wormwood, pumpkin and sesame seeds.

Women lose 15–30 mg iron with each period and as much as 500 mg during childbirth and pregnant women need as much as 120 mg daily. If you are in any doubt about your iron intake from natural sources use the following formula, especially during the last three months of pregnancy.

3 parts yellow dock
1 part gentian
1 part burdock

Take two size 'O' capsules of the finely powdered herbs morning and evening on an empty stomach. Do not drink tea, coffee or chocolate during the time you are taking this formula. Replace them with herbal teas and coffee substitutes – ideally dandelion-root coffee (see Chapter 1).

IODINE

A deficiency of iodine in pregnancy increases the risk of a still-birth and may cause other problems. Pregnant women can safely take as much as 3 mg a day, which should ideally be obtained from safe natural sources by eating nori seaweed or sprinkling a liberal teaspoonful of kelp over every vegetable meal. I'll admit it tastes terrible over cereal, which is why I will let you off at breakfast!

ZINC

This is extremely important to the rapidly growing child in the womb in order to protect her from malformations and an unpleasant skin malfunction.

Zinc is richly present in alfalfa, red raspberry leaves, eyebright, slippery elm, cramp-bark, echinacea and yellow dock, as well as brewer's yeast, seeds, apricots, peaches and dark-green leafy vegetables. It is superabundant in liver. Adequate intake will help prevent stretch marks. Excessive coffee, and elevated levels of copper, calcium and cadmium aggravate low zinc levels. Aim for 30 mg daily.

VITAMIN A

If, during the course of your pregnancy, you suffer from an infection or are exposed to a serious illness like German measles, you will need to take vitamin A in temporarily high doses. Take 50,000 IU, for eight weeks only, in consultation with your doctor. Fat-soluble vitamins have difficulty passing through the placenta, and babies born with a vitamin A deficiency will be particularly susceptible to infection. It is a good idea to drink plenty of carrot juice during the last months of pregnancy as vitamin A from this source is more easily assimilated than that from fatty sources. Fortunately, the colostrum you first feed your baby will contain a particularly plentiful supply of fat-soluble vitamins and will help build up the baby's auto-immune system quickly.

B-COMPLEX VITAMINS

Many of the illnesses common to pregnancy like nausea and oedema are often exacerbated by lack of this group of vitamins, especially B_6. All pregnant and breast-feeding women need 4 mg vitamin B_6 daily but as a therapeutic dose to help morning sickness they can take as much as 300–500 mg daily.

The richest source of the B-complex group (B_6 will not work in isolation) includes brewer's yeast, black strap molasses, malt extract, wheatgerm and its bran, sunflower seeds, soy beans, ground rice, tomatoes, sweetcorn, barley, sweet potatoes, bananas, peanuts and cabbage.

VITAMIN E

The need for this vastly increases during pregnancy, so a supplement is certainly necessary. Your daily dose should be 800–1,000 IU but you cannot start with this much if you have blood-pressure problems, and vitamin E should not be taken as a supplement if there is history of rheumatic fever, over-active thyroid or diabetes. If you get toxaemia you must stop supplementation immediately, so ensure that your blood pressure is checked on a regular basis. Under ordinary circumstances if you are reducing your vitamin E intake do so gently and gradually.

If you are taking iron supplementation, separate this from your vitamin E dose by at least eight hours. D-alpha-tocopherol is the preferred type of vitamin E supplement and is richly present in wholegrains, and seeds and their cold-pressed oils. Eleven per cent is lost if these foods are heated.

VITAMIN K

If the intestinal bacteria are healthy, they generally produce sufficient vitamin K, but because this vitamin is fat-soluble, it cannot easily pass through the placenta into the blood of the foetus. This means that newborn babies are particularly susceptible to haemorrhage as they enter the first week of life. To protect them against this, many obstetricians now inject vitamin K some 20–24 hours before labour begins. Establish in advance that this will be the case because you certainly will not be in a position to do so when you are actually in labour.

Natural sources of vitamin K include kelp, alfalfa, all dark-green leafy vegetables, milk, plain live yoghurt, black strap molasses, apricots, cod-liver oil, sunflower oil and garlic. Supplementation for the baby is not necessary while breast-feeding if the mother's diet is abundant in these foods.

Drugs

Don't take any at all, not even aspirin – use natural alternatives. Drugs cross the placenta and can damage the foetus. Analgesics can prolong pregnancy and labour and lead to severe bleeding in both mother and baby. Anti-acids like bicarbonate of soda can cause muscle problems in the foetus or oedema in the mother. Some cough-mixtures can cause birth defects. Tranquillizers and sedatives can lead to foetal addiction and breathing problems. Tetracycline is deposited in the bones and will lead to poor bone growth. Sulphonamide antibiotics affect the liver and induce kernicterus in newborn babies. (Kernicterus is the result of bilirubin being released into the foetal bloodstream and accumulating in the brain, resulting in permanent brain damage.) Mineral-based laxatives suppress vitamin absorption and can lead to blood disorders in the baby. Even certain chemical-based creams and ointments, such as some of those used for piles, can be absorbed by the placenta and cause deformities. Warfarin can result in undergrowth of the nasal bones and mental retardation. Certain anti-convulsants can cause foetal abnormalities, though a pregnant woman prone to epilepsy must be protected from seizures because they deprive the developing baby of oxygen and so may be even more damaging than the drug. An experienced medical herbalist can help control petit mal forms but this is a complicated business and beyond the scope of this book, so seek professional help. Certain types of grand mal seizures can be helped by sodium-valproate which, so far, seems to be free of any harmful side-effects.

Women on insulin or those who have taken thyroxine for a

long time will need to continue these under close medical supervision. But it is possible to control both thyroid and pancreatic malfunction with herbs and diet, and a far better approach would be to place yourself in the hands of an experienced and qualified medical herbalist well before conception so that you can be gradually weaned onto natural treatment and away from dependency on such drugs. I have succeeded in greatly reducing dependency on thyroxine and insulin with herbal and naturopathic treatment.

Smoking

It is now known that foetal heart-beat can accelerate through anxiety even when the mother is only thinking of having a cigarette. The reduction of oxygen in a baby's blood supply – her only life-line – must be a very unpleasant feeling.

Alcohol

This is rapidly absorbed into the bloodstream and on into the placenta and can stun the baby and make her less active in the womb than she should be. Anyone conceiving after an alcoholic binge is substantially more likely to produce a baby with genetic defects. Even women drinking moderately during pregnancy, say one or two drinks a day, have a much higher chance of miscarriage in mid-term than teetotallers.

Herbs

These need to be strictly controlled in the first three months of pregnancy, and I will never put a pregnant woman through any kind of deep-cleansing programme. Herbs which should not be taken at any time during pregnancy include rue, pennyroyal, oregano, hyssop, myrrh, nutmeg, angelica, mistletoe, juniper, thuja, autumn crocus, barberry, golden-seal, mandrake, male-fern, poke root, tansy, wormwood, southernwood, false unicorn (except to prevent miscarriage), false hellebore and celery seed.

Culinary herbs which should be used only for flavouring in small doses include sage, thyme, basil, savory, marjoram and cinnamon. Blue cohosh is contraindicated except during and just before labour.

Morning Sickness

The fact that morning sickness can often be alleviated by a piece of dry toast or a biscuit suggests hypoglycaemia, although I am convinced that some morning sickness is a result of pre-conceptual inadequate diet. Nausea under the latter circumstances is nature's way of trying to flush the toxins out of the body so that the baby will not be swamped by them. There is some suggestion that increased levels of oestrogen also aggravate morning sickness.

Under all circumstances nausea needs urgent attention if dehydration of the mother is to be avoided, and if it continues into the fourth month should be considered particularly serious.

A diet such as is recommended for hypoglycaemics, eating a little protein every 2–2½ hours, is advisable, and avoiding fatty, spicy and sugary food as well as coffee and alcohol helps. If you decide to try vitamin B_6 supplementation and know you are hypoglycaemic, check with your medical herbalist first as it can also alter blood-sugar levels. Eating a piece of wholewheat toast and sipping a cup of camomile or spearmint tea with ½ teaspoon ginger added before you attempt to get out of bed helps. Some women swear by sucking cherry stones. Or try the following morning-sickness formulation, but do not stay on it too long as prolonged doses of golden-seal may cause the uterus to go into spasms. After a couple of weeks revert to the gingery camomile or spearmint tea instead.

1 part clove
1 part ginger
1 part black horehound
1 part wild yam
½ part golden-seal

Take one size 'O' capsule of the finely powdered herbs on rising and repeat later in the day if necessary.

Cramps

These are generally at their most acute in the last trimester and can be caused by the baby lying awkwardly but more often are the result of a calcium deficiency. They tend to get worse at night as the circulation becomes more laboured. Take 100 mg niacin (to help the circulation) and the calcium formulation (see page 175) with 100 mg vitamin B_6 daily. Vitamin E also helps (see page 178). Sleep with the foot of the bed slightly elevated and use hot foot baths with ten drops of lavender oil added. Drink 1–2 wineglassfuls of cramp-bark decoction daily.

Womb cramping or false labour pains may be treated with a camomile poultice and a daily dose of 1–2 wineglassfuls of cramp-bark decoction taken internally.

Stretch Marks

I have already mentioned zinc supplementation to help with these and Adele Davis also suggests 600 IU vitamin E and 300 mg vitamin B_5 daily. A simple massage oil can be made of 50 mg almond oil, 15 drops of lavender oil and 10 drops of neroli oil. Use it often, applying in gentle circular movements.

Oedema

Vitamin B_6 is helpful here (see page 178), as are hand or footbaths taken twice daily using diuretic herbs like dandelion, garlic, artichoke, hawthorn, birch, cherry, broom and meadow-sweet. Ginger fomentations applied over the kidneys daily are also extremely effective.

Pre-eclampsia

This is serious and must be treated immediately. Symptoms include oedema of the feet, legs, hands and face, hypertension and protein excreted in the urine. In any emergency fast on water melon or boiled brown rice, chew several cloves of raw garlic during the fast and drink a tea made of equal quantities of red clover blossom, ginger, comfrey and dandelion root – 6 wineglassfuls daily. Once the situation is back under control avoid all dairy products, spices, salt, red meat and alcohol and eat an abundance of raw fruit and vegetables.

Varicosity

If you have a family history of low arterial blood pressure you are liable to varicose problems. Nearly a tenth of women get phlebitis or varicose veins during or shortly after pregnancy and this is aggravated by a calcium deficiency, standing for long periods which impedes the circulation, and wearing constricting clothes or shoes. Vitamin E is essential to keep arterial oxygen levels at their optimum; so are foods containing vitamins P and K. Vitamin P (a bioflavonoid otherwise known as rutin, as in buckwheat) needs to be taken as a daily supplement (500 mg) and married up with lecithin (6 teaspoons daily) and plenty of naturally occurring vitamin C.

Exercise helps, especially treading up and down in a bath filled with cold water reaching to the knees for five minutes daily. Also helpful are warm hand and foot baths containing ten drops in all of lavender, garlic or rosemary oil. Use these twice daily. Massaging the legs with 1 fl oz (30 ml) almond oil with four drops of each of cypress and lavender oil and two drops of lemon oil is soothing. Use long, gentle, upward-sweeping strokes. A simple preventative remedy is as follows:

Equal parts of:

Yarrow
stoneroot
cayenne
prickly-ash
lime flowers

Take two size 'O' capsules of the finely powdered herbs with each meal.

Phlebitis

This denotes a clot in the veins of the legs which may result in localized inflammation. Changes in sex hormones in pregnancy cause the blood to clot more readily.

Apply externally fomentations of ice-cold witch-hazel, arnica, comfrey, marigold or hawthorn berries. Raw onion rubbed over the area externally also helps, as does eating garlic (it stops the predisposition to blood clotting). Also take a mixture of the following herbs:

3 parts lime flowers
1 part horsechestnut
1 part buckwheat
1 part yarrow

Take two size 'O' capsules of the finely powdered herbs with a wineglassful of ginger tea with each meal.

Constipation and Diarrhoea

These problems are best treated by short juice fasts (lasting no more than thirty-six hours) and, if the condition is persistent, use of the lower bowel tonic (see page 67). The extra progesterone produced during pregnancy tends to over-relax the intestinal muscles.

Flatulence

Make sure you are not gulping your food. Consider a course of Probion or Superdophilus (see page 64). Take equal parts of finely powdered wild yam and fennel. Three size 'O' capsules with each meal, each dose with a wineglassful of dill or fennel tea.

Miscarriage

The majority of miscarriages occur during the first trimester and are due to foetal abnormalities or a defective implanting of the embryo in the womb. If you are showing any signs of a potential miscarriage, spotting blood for example, telephone your doctor immediately, go and lie down and take Rescue Remedy (see page 137). High doses of vitamins C and E help to prevent miscarriage, as does ensuring that the reproductive organs are strong and non-toxic (see pages 162–3).

Stay in bed and drink ½ cup of the following decoction every half-hour until the bleeding stops, then reduce the dose to hourly every waking hour for three days. Then take one cupful with meals thereafter.

6 parts false unicorn
2 parts squaw vine
2 parts blackcurrant leaves
1 part cramp-bark
1 part wild yam
1 part lobelia
1 part cayenne

The beauty of this combination of herbs is that they will not interfere with the natural process of miscarriage if the foetus is damaged, and if it is dead they will ease its expulsion.

Love-Making During Pregnancy

This is perfectly safe unless there is a risk of miscarriage or unless an ultra-sound scanner shows the placenta to be lying low in the uterus. An orgasm towards the end of pregnancy might set off contractions in the womb strong enough to cause you to go into labour, and some say that prostaglandins found in the semen may bring on labour since the same hormone is used in the tests administered to help induce labour artificially, but to induce labour you will need to use a position where it is injected as high up against the cervix as possible.

Rest assured that the baby is perfectly safe cushioned in her amniotic fluid, so you can be as energetic in your love-making as you like.

Thrush

As you should not douche with anything in pregnancy, simply add one teaspoon of thyme or tea-tree oil to a shallow sitz-bath (see Chapter 6) and bathe in it, letting your knees fall open and splashing the vulva area thoroughly. Avoid all foods containing yeast spores, including vinegar, cider, mushrooms, bread, bought sprouted seeds, malt, cheese, peanuts and pistachio nuts. Also avoid all sugar and dried fruit, as well as tea and coffee.

Easier Delivery

Raspberry (both fruit and leaves) is rich in citrate of iron and tones up the reproductive areas. Mixed in equal quantities with St John's wort, it will help to relieve the after-pains of birth. Massaging the lower back with an essential oil (clary sage, ylang-ylang, rose, neroli or lavender), mixed with a vegetable-oil base, is very helpful. One teaspoon of tincture of black cohosh in water or juice as needed during labour will facilitate a prompt delivery, and if uterine pushing is waning give one size 'O' capsule of golden-seal every half-hour as a safe oxytoxic. Wherever you choose to give birth, check on your doctor's or midwife's attitude to herbs.

Massaging the perineum daily during the last few months of pregnancy with almond or wheatgerm oil will help to prevent tearing.

In Turkey the traditional midwives advise women who have difficult births to drink raw goat's milk – as much as they can – for the last month of pregnancy and during this time to avoid cold water, vinegar and cold food. The milk makes good sense because calcium will help to decrease muscular pain. Some also suggest fasting before the birth, and this may sound extraordinary, but I have known athletes to fast before a big event, swearing that fasting enhances their performance by increasing their stamina and concentration. So fasting (on juices, herbal teas and honey) for a day before labour and of course during labour sounds a reasonable idea (unless you are hypoglycaemic).

My friend Jill Davies used a tincture of equal parts of ginger and cayenne during her recent labour to reduce tension, equalize blood circulation and soothe the nervous system. For my part I went further and added four drops of Rescue Remedy (see page 137) for a labour at which I recently assisted. It should be administered in milk to blunt the fiery taste of the pepper and it can be taken as much or as often as desired. It is certainly wonderfully restorative.

The adrenal formula (see page 172) linked with vitamin B_6 will assist during the prolonged exhausting first stage of labour and will also help the baby, whose adrenal glands are working equally hard. Both the formula and B_6 will also help speed recovery if labour is difficult.

Prenatal formula

This is Dr Christopher's famous formula with which during his lifetime he facilitated many births. It elasticizes the pelvic and vaginal areas, strengthening the reproductive organs for easy delivery.

Equal parts of:

squaw vine
blessed thistle
black cohosh
pennyroyal
false unicorn
raspberry leaves
lobelia

Take two or three size 'O' capsules of the finely powdered herbs morning and evening with a cupful of raspberry leaf or squaw vine tea, beginning six weeks before the birth, *not sooner.*

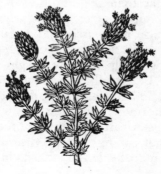

10

Post-natal Care

After-Birth Pain

I have encountered several mothers who have suffered from excessive pain in the coccyx after childbirth and have given them equal parts of tincture of yarrow, arnica and St John's wort (one teaspoon twice daily) with great success.

Feeding

You have heard it before but I will say it again – breast is best. The only medical reason for a baby not being breast-fed is if the mother has active TB, typhoid fever or malaria. Breast milk is germ-free, readily available, requires no preparation and comes at the right temperature. More importantly, it is full of antibodies that protect the baby against disease and immunize her against infections. Breast-fed babies are less likely to suffer from allergies and the lactoferrin in breast milk stops the growth of certain malign yeasts and bacteria in the baby. Breast-fed babies are less likely to become fat than their bottle-fed counterparts, and suckling a baby produces oxytoxin which causes the muscles in the womb to contract and so assists it back into place. There is now a suggestion that breast-feeding lowers the incidence of breast cancer and will help you lose weight and get back into shape more quickly. Breast milk is also lower in salt, and higher in vitamins A and C, and zinc and iron, than cow's milk. It also contains a thyroid hormone which the baby is unable to produce for herself. It has been clearly shown that breast-fed babies have fewer gastrointestinal, ear, respiratory, viral and yeast infections, less meningitis and more benign lactobacilli in their stools.

ALTERNATIVE MILKS

Cow's milk is one of the most common allergy foods. At least 7 per cent of babies are violently allergic to it and many others manifest mild allergy syndrome by way of mucus congestion and diarrhoea. Babies fed cow's milk are more likely to have abnormal calcium and sodium concentrations in their body cells, and to suffer from amino-acid deficiencies, and cot-deaths occur twice as often in babies fed on cow's milk. If you cannot breast-feed you would be better off turning to sheep or goat's milk. The fat content and the size of the fat globules in goat's milk mimic breast milk, and goat's milk is easily digested – in twenty minutes compared to the two hours it takes to process the much larger fatty globules of cow's milk. Soya milk is not rich enough in iron and calcium, and while it can be mixed with goat's or sheep's milk it should not be given on its own. Avoid the sort of soya milk that comes laced with sugar, salt or corn syrup.

MEDICATION WHILE BREAST-FEEDING

The final indisputable advantage of breast milk is that gentle medication for the baby can be given easily and with control by giving the mother herbs – she will transport them in easily digestible form to her baby. I have used in precisely this way heart's-ease and the calcium formula to cure crusta lactaea ('cradle cap'); catnip and fennel to soothe colic; camomile to soothe digestive upsets; and tormentil for diarrhoea.

Do remember that alcohol, nicotine, caffeine, opiates, tranquillizers, quinine, antibiotics and laxatives, as well as vitamin C, all pass through into breast milk in small amounts. Barbiturates, aspirin, iodine, bromides and ergot all flood into breast milk copiously.

So if you need antibiotics while breast-feeding take the following natural alternative. A tincture made of equal parts of:

butterbur
nasturtium
horseradish
watercress
Garden Cress

Put 40 drops in a cup of water and take a teaspoon every fifteen minutes while the infection is acute. Reduce to 10 drops (taken in water) three times daily if it is persistent. This is Dr Vogal's remedy, commercially available under the name of Petroconale.

Boost the baby's auto-immune system by including in your diet lots of the herbs that fight bacteria – thyme, sage, garlic, rosemary, marigold. If you have never thought of eating the latter, try sprinkling the petals over salads or baking them into bread – pretty and tasty with it.

COLOSTRUM
This starts being produced after the sixteenth week of pregnancy, and by the thirtieth week can be expressed by hand to encourage the milk ducts to open. It will come out in drops of thick yellow fluid and is abundantly present in the first three or four days after birth. It is higher in protein, vitamin A and minerals than later breast milk and lower in carbohydrates and fats. Its reduced fat content makes it easier to digest. It is also mildly laxative, which helps the baby clear her digestive tract of meconium (the early greenish-black stools that accumulate while in the uterus). Like mature breast milk, colostrum contains antibodies against bacteria and viruses. These antibodies slow or stop the growth of flu, encephalitis, polio, mumps and *E. coli*. The long-term reward of colostrum followed by breast milk is a resoundingly healthy colon for the baby later in life.

DIET WHILE BREAST-FEEDING
Nursing mothers actually need more protein and calories than they needed in the last trimester and calorie content should be as high as 2,600 daily. Vitamins A, C and B_{12} as well as iodine and iron all need to be increased. Juliette de Bairacli-Levy recommends a restorative drink of 1 dessertspoon of a mixture of cloves, cinnamon and candied ginger pounded up and added to a pint of sweet white wine as a restorative drink immediately after labour. Other mothers may prefer raspberry-leaf tea with lots of honey, cloves, cinnamon and ginger added.

QUALITY AND FLOW
Good milk is thin and flows easily. It should smell good, be pure (almost bluish) white in colour and taste sweet. To test your milk, put a little on your fingernail and tilt the finger upwards. If the milk does not trickle down easily it is too thick. Herbs which

improve the quality of milk are marshmallow and borage. Try the very young leaves of borage as a delicious alternative to cucumber in your salads; and the beautiful blue flowers can be used in the same way. Herbs which increase the flow of breast milk are fennel, cinnamon, anise, blessed thistle, vervain, fenugreek, goat's-rue and caraway.

To thin breast milk

Drink 2 fl oz (60 ml) cider vinegar mixed with a tablespoon honey in hot water twice daily, and eat lots of hyssop, thyme and borage. If you can get them fresh, sprinkle them in foods and cook with them, but dried herbs are also acceptable. In this case make teas of them.

To thicken breast milk

Eat lots of soupy grains (such as green lentils and orange lentils), and lace them liberally with plenty of garlic and onions. Add plenty of sage, blessed thistle, comfrey and red clover blossom to the diet. The flowers of red clover make an unusual addition to salads in the summer.

SORE NIPPLES

Pound up a handful of fresh lady's-mantle leaves until they are finely mulched, or hydrate a tablespoon of the dried leaves by soaking them for twenty minutes in just enough hot water to cover. Stir in enough honey to form a thick poultice and spread this over the nipple. Cover it with gauze, a square of plastic and a soft nursing bra. Keep the nipples supple by oiling them or applying a little buttermilk or honey.

INABILITY TO PRODUCE MILK

False unicorn mixed with other galactagogues (substances that promote milk secretion) is believed to encourage the flow of breast milk. Certainly a baby's frequent sucking action helps. I am also told that Sicilian women who have never had babies sometimes induce a flow of milk by putting drops of goat's milk onto the nipple whenever the baby is about to give up sucking at the non-productive breast. After persisting with this for two weeks, their own milk begins to flow. It is worth a try if you are apparently unable to breast-feed but very much want to do so.

WEANING

The comfort of breast-feeding is not easily forgone by the baby, so wean her gently and gradually. Drink large amounts of cold red-sage tea to dry up your milk, and if the baby is fretful and insists on the breast, make a poultice of 1 oz (30 g) freshly ground, finely milled pennyroyal mixed with equal quantities of myrrh. Mix with a little purified water and spread over the nipples. You will notice that when the baby sucks on this she rapidly loses her desire to suckle. But it makes coming off the breast less traumatic for her.

Fatigue

It is often fatigue that swamps new parents, due to stress, lack of sleep and extra work, once they have come down off the initial euphoria. So take catnaps during the day as soon as the baby sleeps; go to sleep very early at night initially; reduce visitors; aim for one hour's complete relaxation daily doing something that is purely pleasurable for yourself; do not be afraid to seek help from friends; make sure that both you and your partner get optimum nutrition. Above all, be determined not to get overwhelmed by your new responsibilities and do not get anxious. The chances of your baby suddenly becoming extremely ill or manifesting a hidden abnormality in the days after the birth are very remote. Babies are built to survive!

Bathing Yourself and Your Baby

If you can bear it, as soon as possible after the birth take alternating cold and hot sitz-baths (see Chapter 6) every morning and evening. Add a teaspoon of thyme oil to each bath and practise your PC exercises (see Chapter 9) in the bath. If the perineum is swollen, use lavender oil instead and apply a few drops diluted in wheatgerm oil directly, wearing a panty liner to protect knickers. If you have had an episiotomy, apply a poultice of fresh comfrey leaves or the powdered root, and as soon as the cut shows signs of healing start to massage vitamin E oil and St John's wort oil into it. Avoid constipation at all costs. You may have to resort to sitting on a rubber ring – undignified but effective. Cold sitz-baths will speed the discharge of lochia and encourage the womb to shrink back to its normal size as well as tone up the pelvic-floor muscles. In Kenya, my ayah told me, it is customary for the midwife to massage the abdomen to get the body back into shape but this is obviously a special skill. To firm your breasts, use a forceful cold shower on them after a warm bath.

It can be frightening washing a tiny newborn baby in a bath as they tend to feel very slippery. Frequent baths taken at blood heat encourage skin activity, remove congestion and stimulate the internal organs and lymphatic system. Do not use soap. A bag of oatmeal is preferable, followed with a dash of cider vinegar in the bath water to restore the baby's acid mantle. An infusion of lady's-mantle added to bath water will help with any tendency to hernia; camomile is good for digestive and metabolic disturbances; marigold for skin rashes; wild thyme to protect against colds; and lemon balm works wonders on fractious babies.

Massaging the whole body with St John's wort oil works better than powder to protect against nappy rash and is a good antiseptic. Avoid oil only if the baby has infant acne. Massaging yourself with equal parts of ylang-ylang, lavender and marjoram in a carrier base of almond oil is wonderfully soothing. Do not forget that you need mothering every bit as much as your baby.

Love-making

As you pour your initial attention into the baby and take time to heal yourself, your libido will be understandably low. But once you feel comfortable and enthused again you must think seriously about contraception. Even if you breast-feed, it is by no means impossible to conceive within the first 4–6 weeks following birth. Admittedly it is unusual for a woman to menstruate within twenty-eight days of delivery and most nursing mothers do not ovulate for twenty-two weeks after delivery.

Post-natal Depression

This has now reached virtually epidemic proportions in this country. It seems that one in ten mothers suffer from it, and the disease is so widely recognized that if a woman kills her baby within twelve months of its birth, the crime is not 'murder' – the term used instead is 'infanticide'. Post-natal depression can drag on for as much as a year, and one of my patients likened it to permanently having flu. The problem has been variously attributed to hormonal imbalance and a lack of progesterone as well as high levels of stress, changes in lifestyle and social status, immediate separation from the baby after birth, an unexpected caesarean, or over-sedation during the birth. Whatever the combination of causes, communication is vital. There is an association specifically set up to help with this problem (see Appendix).

Keep your diet optimal and take 9 g vitamin C daily, and twice daily a strong B-complex supplement with 75 mg of each B fraction in it.

Equal parts of:

lemon balm
gota kola
pasque-flower
Cornsilk
lady's-slipper
scullcap
vervain

Take three size 'O' capsules of the finely powdered herbs with every meal. Do your skin-scrubbing and barefoot walking morning and evening. Force yourself to. Depression can be greatly alleviated by purposeful action. Lean on those you love for support. They will be glad you did.

11

The Menopause

The menopause is another very important rite of passage. No comparable phenomenon takes place in a man's body. Men can remain fertile throughout their lives, and although testosterone levels drop they continue to produce viable new sperm. The menopause is a good time to pause, literally; to rest for a moment and re-examine your values, to enjoy your accomplishments and most of all to love and appreciate your female processes. It is a beginning not an ending; a time for looking forward, not one of sadness or regret; a time for a renewal, not for a fear of ageing. Paavo Airola puts it beautifully:

Menopause is a divinely designed phase in a woman's life, with the purpose of liberating her from duties as pro-creator with God and giving her time for self-improvement, for the perfection of her human and divine characteristics, and her spiritual growth.

Actually the first signs of ageing begin long before the menopause. The lenses of the eyes begin to deteriorate at the age of ten. Hearing the upper frequencies starts to become more difficult at the same age. Certainly the body's ability to repair itself is declining by the age of forty, and at this time the pressure of weight on the spinal column begins to take its toll, actually decreasing height; but bones can be strengthened and their shrinkage stopped by exercise. The thyroid shrinks, slowing down metabolic rate and signalling a subsequent decline in other hormones. Within the first two years of the menopause three-quarters of ovarian oestrogen production is lost, but some of the ovaries' work is taken over by the adrenals. If the adrenals have been exhausted by an overactive sympathetic nervous system, poor nutrition or a malfunctioning liver or heart, they are incapable of taking on this extra workload. So healthy adrenal glands are a prerequisite to a comfortable menopause and the formula on page 172 will help here.

The good news is that intelligence and memory remain intact, and that many of the other symptoms of ageing can be alleviated, slowed or checked by a superabundance of vitamins, minerals and enzymes in a particularly conscientious diet. This includes the rigorous avoidance of anything with chemicals in it, as well as meat, tea and coffee, and sugar, and extreme moderation with alcohol. Fertile eggs, yoghurt and buttermilk should be the nearest you get to an animal.

Eating less and, particularly, fasting actively slow down the ageing process and accelerate the repair processes in the body. I undertake one long fast yearly, usually a three-week one, and several shorter ones of 4–7 days and they are times of self-pleasuring I keenly anticipate.

Natural hormones are abundantly available in certain foods and herbs. Never forget the importance of adequate rest and correct breathing – one of the most vital women I ever met was an eighty-year-old yoga teacher who swore by her 'vitamins of the air'. Yoga itself helps to keep the body supple. Stiffness and pain are not natural concomitants of ageing. When I was in China I saw sixty- and seventy-year-old women practising t'ai chi with a grace, suppleness and beauty that would have shamed many of our degenerate thirty-year-olds.

Avoiding Hormone Replacement Therapy

Too many of my patients come to me believing that their menopausal discomforts can be relieved by synthetic oestrogen and find, to their disappointment, that the moment that they stop taking it the symptoms reassert themselves in no uncertain terms. This is because hormone replacement therapy is too often used prophylactically to prevent symptoms. The truth is that really healthy women seldom experience menopausal difficulties. So the secret of a trouble-free menopause is to get yourself into really good shape well before it starts.

In this country oestrogen and progestogen are prescribed in a pattern that mimics a woman's hormonal output during the menopausal cycle, but synthetic oestrogen increases the need for vitamin E; and even Premarin, fondly billed as the 'natural' form of oestrogen (presumably because it is collected from the urine of mares) is just as capable of causing dangerous blood clots as the synthetic oestrogen. Gall-stones are much more common among women who take hormone replacement therapy, and it is definitely not advisable for those with high blood pressure, a past history of thrombosis of any kind, diabetes, or chronic liver disease, or for smokers or those with a family history of heart disease.

I feel very strongly that manmade chemicals are bad for the body and this includes synthetic hormones. Foods which are particularly rich in natural hormones include seeds and sprouted seeds, wholegrains, royal jelly, bee pollen, bananas, carrots, potatoes, apples, cherries, plums and garlic.

Wholegrain porridge
This is a delicious hormone-rich way to start the day which insures maximum food value because the grains are pre-soaked and only subjected to low heat and therefore retain their entire nutritional value, unlike the ground-up grains you use for baking.

Early in the evening fill a wide-necked thermos flask one third full with whole buckwheat, whole millet, whole wheat, whole oats or whole barley. Fill the rest of the flask with boiling water. Seal. Shake and leave overnight. When you open the flask the next morning the grains will have popped open and be softly chewy and very tasty. Serve with a little unsalted butter, together with honey, maple syrup, ginger or cinnamon, and add pre-soaked dried fruit or a well-ripened banana. Sprinkle in equal parts of sunflower seeds, sesame seeds and pumpkin seeds. Do not let the temperature exceed 130°F (54°C). If you want to find out just how 'live' the grain still is, save a little and watch it sprout.

Oestrogen-rich formula
Equal parts of:

  false unicorn
  liquorice
  blessed thistle
  raspberry

wild yam
sage
lady's slipper
pasque-flower
elderflowers
lobeli

Alternatively use the formula on page 163. Take two size 'O' capsules of the finely powdered herbs with a cup of sarsaparilla tea with each meal. Both these formulae will help after a hysterectomy and are generally beneficial throughout the menopause.

Hot Flushes

During a hot flush the skin is suddenly suffused with blood and turns bright red, inducing sweating and heat. It helps to wear layers of clothing so that you can peel a few off if a flush overwhelms you. It seems that a certain level of oestrogen must be present in the blood for hot flushes to occur because flushes are rare in pre-menopausal women and even more so in post-menopausal ones. This 'flushing band' is narrower in some women than others but most women experience it, even if only for a few months. In some it goes on for years, and when it happens at night, enforcing several changes of bedding, it can be a particularly miserable experience.

Take the following formula on the days hot flushes occur and revert to the one on pages 144-5 on the other days.

2 parts rosemary
1 part spearmint
1 part mugwort
1 part St John's wort
1 part vervain
1 part false unicorn

Take one size 'O' capsule of the finely powdered herbs every two hours with sips of sage tea. Also take hand baths made with equal parts of mistletoe leaves, sage, hawthorn and vine leaves.

Night Sweats

A very simple but effective solution that I have found to work extremely well with my own patients is 3 drops of essential oil of sage taken with honey and hot water just before bed.

Excessively Heavy Periods

The normal course of the menopause is for menstruation to become erratic with longer and longer gaps between periods, or simply for periods to become lighter and shorter until they eventually stop. Sometimes menstruation will stop suddenly once and for all but this is very rare.

Please note that it is never normal to have frequent heavy periods or to pass blood clots during the menopause. Pain, spotting in-between periods and after love-making are equally unacceptable. In an emergency if you are haemorrhaging, use a warm infusion of cayenne as a douche and put 1 teaspoon cayenne in a cup of warm water, drinking it quickly. But consult your doctor immediately.

Vaginal Changes

The inside of the vagina is lined with flattened mucous epithelial cells, some thirty deep, that are continually shed, rather like skin cells. In the case of the vagina, harmless resident bacteria help decompose the cell detritus and in doing so manufacture lactic acid, which protects the vagina against harmful bacteria. Hence the vagina is generally able to look after itself without much conscious help. But as oestrogen levels fall the vagina changes dramatically. The cells of the lining thin, dry out and are unable to fend off invading bacteria, so offensive vaginal discharges are much more common during the menopause and afterwards. The subsequent pain with love-making can naturally put a woman off sex. The synthetic hormone creams do nothing to restore the vagina to its former state, and remember that such creams are easily absorbed into the bloodstream. Vitamin E taken internally and used externally in vaginal boluses (using cocoa butter as a base) helps, as does KY jelly or saliva. The good news is that frequent intercourse keeps the vagina youthful. It seems that lubrication has much less to do with the intensity of stimulation than with its duration, so if you find yourself getting into difficulties, share this invaluable piece of information with your partner. However, experimenting with such advice must be done gently. In the post-menopausal woman whose clitoris is relatively more exposed because of labial atrophy, this exquisitely sensitive area will become more vulnerable to direct stimulation during intercourse. Any stimulation which is too intense far from being exciting can be distressing and painful.

Sexual Response in the Menopause

Vaginal lubrication may wane but your ability to respond during love-making certainly does not. Some women, freed from the risks of getting pregnant, profess to enjoy sex even more. It may take longer to reach the plateau phase of sexual excitement but this applies equally to men. The signs of a plateau phase dwindle. The labia minora do not darken so much, and the labia majora are less inclined to swell, but the clitoral response remains as vigorous as ever. The intensity and duration of orgasm tend to decrease but the ability to have multiple orgasms continues. So overall if your sex life was enjoyable before the menopause it will probably continue to be so afterwards – particularly if your partner is able to prolong and enhance foreplay.

Prolapse of the Uterus

This generally happens because of problems during delivery – either the delivery is too rapid or the second stage of labour is too prolonged. Stretching and tearing can occur either way, or it can be caused by forceps delivery if forceps are used when the baby's head is still very high. Less commonly, strenuous physical activity can result in a prolapse.

Initial symptoms are a feeling of dragging down in the pelvis; backache; incontinence on coughing, laughing, sneezing or jumping; an uncomfortable feeling during love-making because of the pressure from organs bearing downwards; and lack of vaginal tone.

The exercises on page 171 will help, as will maintaining a normal weight.

Herbal injection for prolapse
You will need to administer this while lying on a slant board with a pillow placed underneath the hips to raise them. Alternatively, if you are really fit you can hold the liquid while in a shoulder stand. Make a decoction of:

6 parts oak barn
6 parts comfrey root
4 parts yellow dock
3 parts lady's mantle
3 parts marshmallow root
1 part St John's wort
1 part nettles

Strain thoroughly. Cool. On rising in the morning inject ¼–1 cup of the decoction into the vagina with a douche kit (see page 124) and hold it for 5–10 minutes. Expel it. Repeat before retiring. Also drink a wineglassful of the decoction morning and evening with meals. If the prolapse is very severe, inject the same amount into the rectum immediately after the vaginal injection and hold both simultaneously for the same length of time. This treatment needs to be kept up faithfully for many months before you can expect any improvement.

Depression

The bedrock of depression is a feeling of not being in control of one's life, a sense of powerlessness. The problem is that society sets women up for depression by strait-jacketing many of them into the role of wife and mother. Very few women even today are completely financially independent. As they grow older they tend to become more dependent if not on their husbands then on their children, not simply for money but for companionship, care in ill health and transportation. Add to this physical problems during the menopause, some of which can be quite debilitating, and it is not surprising that depression is often exacerbated at this time of life.

Physical exercise helps, as does a close examination of one's attitude towards ageing and towards one's place in society. I often cite to patients who need steering in the right direction the example of my favourite adopted aunt. As her children left home and her husband became increasingly immersed in his own burgeoning career she could have sat at home moping and feeling useless. Instead she pushed herself against the system that conditioned her to see herself in terms of marriage, children and housekeeping and carved out a new role for herself by going back to school and working her way right through from 'O' levels to a teaching qualification. She is now a very expert and fulfilled remedial teacher. And she looks more lively and more beautiful than I remember her twenty years ago.

The following nervine formula is helpful.

Equal parts of:

rosemary
blue vervain
raspberry
hops
valerian
lady's-slipper

Take one size 'O' capsule of the finely powdered herbs every waking hour as needed, and once the worst of the depression is over reduce the dose to the two capsules three times daily with meals.

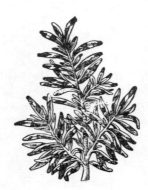

12

Problems

If I could have only one wish it would be to live in a world like this one, at a time like the present, enjoying all the friends and the problems I have now, and above all to be myself in this world. 'Enjoying' problems may seem a decidedly strange concept but I have always felt that all serious setbacks, including illness, are given to us as ideal opportunities to learn about ourselves and our place in the world, chemically, nutritionally, biologically, spiritually, socially, and emotionally. Approached in that spirit illness can revolutionize your life.

When I was twenty-one I had a nervous breakdown, and because I didn't take on board the lessons I should have learned from it I had another when I was twenty-six. The second time around I was a bit wiser and, gradually, in spite of the pain of it, I began to learn the reasons why and, more importantly, how to help myself and how to ensure it never happened again. But I have never regretted the illness. Not only was it an invaluable lesson about my own Achilles' heel, stress, but it has since enabled me both to empathize with and to help other women in the same position.

As Somerset Maugham observed, 'It is a funny thing about life: if you refuse to accept anything but the best, you very often get it.' So put illness in this positive context and see it as an opportunity not just for struggle and pain but for enlightenment and growth, as an ideal means to build on strengths and understand weaknesses.

Depression

The mentally ill occupy more than a third of all National Health Service beds. You are more likely to suffer from depression if any of the following factors apply: isolation, no close friends to confide in, having no work outside the home, poor housing, bad financial problems, looking after toddlers at home full-time, and losing your mother at an early age. The roots of depression spring from not being in control of one's life. Feminist sociologist Pauline Bart defines depression as a response to powerlessness. She believes that society sets women up for depression by encouraging or forcing them to put 'all their eggs in one or at the most two baskets – the mother role and the wife role'. Many women when they lose either of these roles respond with a loss of identity and a sense of powerlessness and uselessness.

REMEDIES FOR DEPRESSION

Fighting back helps. If your rights or dignity are being trampled on summon the energy to stand up for yourself. Say what you mean. Show your feelings. Purposeful activity helps – ensure that it is something you enjoy and will give you a sense of accomplishment.

One of the most common physical signs of depression is fatigue. Exercise helps. Make it regular, vigorous and enjoyable, and – given time – it will revolutionize your physical and mental well-being.

Anxiety

Valium is the largest-selling prescriptive drug sold in the world today and women users outnumber men by a very large margin. 'Anxiety' is such a loose definition of a wide range of physical symptoms that anti-anxiety drugs can be prescribed for virtually any reason (and judging by the number of my patients who take them very often are). Physical symptoms of stress apart from fatigue may include weakness; sweating; trembling; breathlessness; choking; fainting; hypertension; palpitations; digestive upsets; over-dependence on alcohol, drugs or tobacco; loss of interest in sex; insomnia; or simply a succession of mysterious aches, pains and niggling little discomforts. Allopathic prescriptions merely mask the symptoms and do nothing to deal with the social, emotional and physical conditions which are the cause.

It is now well known that anti-anxiety drugs are addictive, and here herbs can play an invaluable part in helping a patient to withdraw from them – coupled with counselling, a good diet, plenty of exercise, the support of friends, and stress-management techniques like meditation, yoga, self-hypnosis, visualization, autogenics or biofeedback. A prolonged dose of any of the benzodiazepines will produce withdrawal symptoms if stopped, and I have observed that some very sensitive patients experience the same symptoms on smaller, shorter-term doses. Withdrawal symptoms include anxiety, dysphoria and occasionally con-vulsions and severe emotional and perceptive changes such as seeing glittering lights, unsteadiness and experiencing noises and sensations of motion while resting.

Weaning long-term users off Ativan, Serenid and Euhypnos, which are stronger, is harder than getting people of Librium, Valium, Mogadon, Dalmane and Tranxene, but herbal remedies will act as a useful bridge as the dosages of the chemical medicines are very slowly and gently reduced. Herbs will actively tone, strengthen and nourish a battered nervous system which has hitherto been exposed to the heavy chemical stress of allopathic tranquillizers. Both valerian and scullcap initially replace the benzodiazepine's effect while strengthening the nervous system, so helping to ease withdrawal symptoms. They are not rec-ommended for long-term use. Camomile, catnip, hops, lavender, lemon balm, lime flowers, mistletoe, pasque-flower, red clover, rosemary, vervain, motherwort, woodruff, oats and the ginsengs all have a useful part to play as adaptogens or for the broad support the body needs during the process of withdrawal.

If you have been taking any of the allopathic tranquillizers for longer than two months it is unwise to try and wean yourself off them without the support and advice of a qualified medical herbalist.

Nerve tonic
Equal parts of:

> black cohosh
> hops
> lady's-slipper
> scullcap
> lobelia

valerian
wood betony
hawthorn
mistletoe
mugwort
lemon balm
ginger

Make a tincture and take 2–3 teaspoons three times daily, preferably stirred into a hot drink.

Vaginal Secretions and Infections

A lot of women on the Pill do not appreciate what normal vaginal secretions should look like because the Pill tends to distort or diminish them. Tiny, clear droplets of fluid form on the walls of the vagina and mix with the sloughed-off cells, which give the secretions a white appearance. The cervical canal secretes a thicker mucus, which can be either clear or white, and this too flows into the vagina. Vaginal secretions are usually slightly acid, whereas cervical secretions are also slightly acid when whitish non-fertile mucus is being secreted but are alkaline when secretions are fertile and clear. The abundance of secretions varies from woman to woman. Some have heavy secretions throughout the menstrual cycle. Others notice an increase in secretions around ovulation which can actually wet the crotch of knickers, while others, especially those on the Pill, have very little secretion at any time of the month.

A healthy vagina can be besieged by many irritants. Resistance to infection can be reduced by stress, drugs, poor general health, or irritation to the membranes of the vulva, vagina and clitoris. Tight clothing, synthetic fibres, vigorous or prolonged coitus, diaphragms, an IUD string, condoms, tampons, spermicidal creams, deodorant sprays, bubble baths and soap, vibrators and douche solutions can all cause irritation and leave you vulnerable to infection. A prolapsed colon, poor pelvic muscle tone and a sloppy diet can also result in infection.

The odour of a discharge is an important clue in identifying an infection. All of us have a certain amount of vulval odour which smells pleasantly musky as opposed to the sour, strong, often fishy smell of a yeast discharge or the pronounced fetid odour of a bacterial infection. Yeast infections are usually heavy, thick, curdy and white, occasionally tinged with grey or green, while bacterial infections tend to be brownish and runny. It is important to realize that it is possible to have more than one infection at a time. Trichomonas often accompanies the greenish-yellow discharge of gonorrhea, for example.

THRUSH

Also called moniliasis, candidiasis or yeast infection, this is caused by a fungus, *Candida albicans*, that only produces problems when it multiplies and changes its form. It thrives in a moist, warm environment (so is particularly prevalent in hot, humid weather), can be spread by sharing bathing suits or towels, can live under the foreskin of the penis, and can be transmitted during love-making. It loves refined carbohydrates and sugar, and is precipitated by antibiotics (see page 62); and many women on oral contraceptives are more prone to thrush because these contraceptives promote a sweeter vaginal environment, encouraging fungal growth. The infection manifests itself as vaginal itching and may result in a thick, curdy discharge and possible pain on urination.

If the itching is unbearable, make a poultice of slippery elm and golden seal, adding a touch of cider vinegar when mixing. Spread this in a thick paste over the vulva and labia and secure it in position with a sanitary towel. Douche once daily with motherwort and golden seal tea mixed with 1 tablespoon cider vinegar, retaining the douche as long as possible. A steeply raised slant board or a shoulder stand are both positions that will help here. Before bed insert two Probion tablets as deeply into the vagina as possible. Take these orally too (see Appendix). After washing, pat-dry with a clean towel and wipe with pure olive oil if not using the slippery elm poultice. Avocado and olive oil contain oleic acid which prevents the yeast from proliferating.

Remedy for thrush
Equal parts of:

  echinacea
  golden seal

periwinkle
squaw vine
garlic

Take one size 'O' capsule of the finely powdered herbs hourly with sips of oatstraw tea until the yeast infection is under control; then reduce to two with each meal.

The course of herbs should last for at least twenty-eight days in all. Your partner must also be treated with equal parts of echinacea, golden seal, garlic and marshmallow: two size 'O' capsules with each meal for the duration of your course of treatment. This will ensure that the infection is not passed back and forth.

LEUCORRHOEA
This is called 'the whites' because it shows itself as a white vaginal discharge which causes itchiness and pain. Fast for three days on vegetable juices only and take half a cup of the following tea hourly:

2 parts blue flag
2 parts sage
1 part parsley
1 part echinacea
1 part dandelion
1 part golden seal
½ part cinnamon

Douche twice daily with equal parts of golden seal, sage and comfrey, adding a tablespoon of cider vinegar to the mix and retaining the douche as long as possible.

BACTERIAL INFECTIONS
Infections which are neither yeast nor trichomonas are called non-specific vaginitis. Bacterial infections can be caused by the over-growth of bacteria, which travel from an infection in the urinary tract or the intestinal tract to the vagina. They can be passed on during love-making if your partner has a urethral infection, or after anal intercourse if the penis is not washed before vaginal insertion. Multiplication of bacteria will cause pain, itching and a runny, foul-smelling, usually brown discharge.

Douche with equal parts of comfrey, sage, golden-seal and camomile with a tablespoon of cider vinegar added. Do this twice daily for no more than seven consecutive days.

Take the antibiotic on page 189 for three consecutive weeks.

TRICHOMONAS

These tiny one-celled creatures are always with us and only become a problem when they get out of hand and multiply. Their origin is unknown but they are usually transmitted by sexual contact – more specifically, a woman usually acquires them from under the foreskin of a penis or from a man's urethra or prostate gland. Ninety per cent of the partners of women suffering from trichomonas are infected with it too. Rarely, lesbians can transmit trichomonas, and very occasionally it can be passed from moist objects like towels, flannels or toilet seats.

Trichomonas has a tendency to recur the week after menstruation, so douching for the whole week during this time with 1 tablespoon golden-seal tincture and 1 teaspoon tincture of myrrh diluted in 3½ pints (2 litres) water is particularly helpful. Men should wash under their foreskin with this solution and wear a condom for three months when making love. Inserting a clove of garlic (peeled but without nicking the garlic flesh with the knife or fingernail) as high up into the vaginal canal as possible nightly is also helpful. If you are worried about not being able to retrieve it, wrap the clove in a piece of gauze 12 in (30 cm) long and 1 in (2.5 cm) wide. Fold this in half and twist it just below the clove, making a small tampon with a long tail. Dip the clove end in olive oil and insert. Change twice daily.

Cystitis

This manifests itself in a frequent and urgent need to urinate and a burning pain on doing so. Sometimes the urine is blood-stained and there may be pain in the lower abdomen, and mild fever.

Cystitis is often assumed to be the result of a bacterial infection, but in about 50 per cent of cases no sign of infection can be traced, and conversely bacteria can often be found in the urine of symptom-free women. It is well known that nervous, anxious women suffer more from cystitis than their mentally stalwart sisters.

Drink a gallon (4.5 litres) of liquid daily and make most of that water. Avoid alcohol and spicy foods. Wash the genitals with a shower-head or over a bidet, and shower don't bath. Do not use soap at all on the genitals. Simply pat dry with a soft towel. Use cotton underwear only, and wash it in pure soap, rinsing it really well. Avoid tight clothing. Don't make love on a full bladder and urinate immediately afterwards to flush out any bacteria that may have crept into the urethra. Occasionally, cystitis may be the result of a food allergy, so a meticulous diet diary helps here.

If you can feel an attack coming on, fast for three days on vegetable juices and warm vegetable broths, as well as barley water and plenty of cranberry juice. Take as much as you can manage of the following infusion – and not less than four cups daily:

4 parts marshmallow
1 part dandelion
1 part cleavers
1 part horsetail
1 part borage
½ part lobelia
½ part ginger

Apply hot fomentations of wild thyme with a pinch of ginger added over the abdomen.

Contact Dermititis of the Vulva

This seems to be on the increase, judging from the patients I see in my practice. Initially it shows itself as a slight reddening of the vulva with itching, but if not treated this can lead to labial swelling and the onset of clear blisters which eventually burst and crust over.

Begin by checking that you are not reacting to something that comes into contact with the vulva – this includes coloured toilet paper, soap, bath additives, soap powder, condoms, vaginal contraceptive foams, tights, feminine sprays, the ingredients in commercial vaginal douches, sanitary towels, and vibrators.

Allergic reaction to aspirin, sulphur drugs, phenacetin and some laxatives may also cause vulval inflammation. Eliminate the offending agents.

Some women get relief from a hot sitz-bath containing a tablespoon of arrowroot, others from cold compresses of a strained decoction of golden seal or of aloe vera juice. Aloe vera ointment is often soothing. Pat, don't rub dry, or use a hairdryer turned on to cool, and dust with arrowroot once dry. Alternatively, use 3 teaspoons almond oil and 1 teaspoon wheatgerm oil, mixed with one drop of lavender oil and one drop of geranium oil, spreading this over the affected area. Once the condition begins to clear, let as much air get to the vulva as possible – hence the ingenious idea of the hairdryer. In the meantime, don't wear tights, or tight-fitting or nylon underwear. Go for loose cotton knickers instead.

Genital Herpes

Cold sores on the mouth are classified as the herpes simplex virus type I. A closely related virus, herpes simplex virus type II, can affect the vulva, cervix and upper vagina. The distinction between the two viruses lies mainly in the areas they infect, but many scientists now feel that differences between types I and II are diminishing.

Anyone who is a cold-sore sufferer will know that they may be quiescent for long periods but will re-emerge under certain predictable conditions – after sunbathing, when a cold is coming, when the sufferer is under stress or around menstruation.

Most genital herpes is caused by contact with a type II virus and is picked up during sexual intercourse. But it is possible to transmit the type I virus from a cold sore from the mouth to the genitals during oral sex. Type I virus is not implicated in the development of cervical cancer (as Type II is), but the physical symptoms can be just as upsetting as those of Type II. They may begin with a fever, swollen and tender lymph nodes, excruciating itching, and painful blisters along the vulva, and graduate to inflammation around the urethral area, making urination excessively painful. In infections with herpes virus type II the cervix may become red, irritated and ulcerated, resulting in discharge and vaginal spotting. If you have had no previous encounter with any of the other herpes viruses, like shingles or cold sores, you will not have acquired appropriate antibodies. Under these circumstances getting herpes virus type II can be very bad news.

The first experience of herpes in the genital area may result in pain on urination or defecation, and a general feeling of malaise – headaches, swollen glands and fever – as well as the more obvious lesions. Such symptoms are an interaction between the virus and host and it is the individual's defence mechanisms which determine how violent and widespread the symptoms are. So it is vital to improve the immune system, thereby robbing the virus of a chance to be active.

ACTIVATING THE VIRUS

Rubbing or chafing the skin, injury, physical or mental stress, sunburn, fever, a poor diet, excessive anger, anxiety, depression and menstruation can all spark viral activity again. An outbreak can last for a couple of days or as much as three weeks.

If a baby comes into contact with active lesions during the process of birth she will also certainly be infected. If there are not active viral lesions normal birth is usually safe, but if there are a caesarean is absolutely necessary.

TREATMENT OF HERPES

Raising the level of the immune system is a prerequisite (see pages 35–9), as is a dietary strategy which involves the reduction of the amino-acid arginine and the simultaneous boosting of lysine, which will help to control the duplication of the viral particles. The foods which are rich in lysine include chicken, lamb, beans, brewer's yeast and beansprouts, as well as most fruits and vegetables except peas. Foods high in arginine are gelatin, chocolate, carob, coconut, oats, wholewheat or white flour, wheatgerms, peanuts and soya beans.

While symptom-free take 0.5–1.5 g lysine daily. When the virus is showing signs of activity increase the dose to 3 g daily. Also take vitamin C and bioflavonoids to saturation point, stopping just short of diarrhoea; and B_5, B_6, folic acid, calcium and magnesium.

Follow all the practical advice given for cystitis concerning soap, water, air and clothes. If pain during urination is excruciating, spraying cold water onto the vulval area from the shower-head while urinating will help. Otherwise sit in a bowl of cold water while urinating. Cold yoghurt compresses applied for ten minutes at a time six times daily over the affected area give some relief. Rinse with a cold shower afterwards and pat on the following tincture.

Equal parts of:

golden seal
scullcap
garlic
lobelia

Patients complain that this stings but say that it is preferable to the constant painful itching. Also take 60 drops of the above tincture in a little water three times daily with meals. Massaging the lymph glands and lower back with 2 fl oz (60 ml) olive oil, 10 drops rose oil and 15 drops lavender oil will help to stimulate the immune system, as will regular lavender baths.

All women who contract genital herpes should have a cervical smear at least once yearly, and be honest with any prospective sexual partner. The fact that the ignorant public still tend to see herpes as the penalty for sexual freedom has led to unnecessary feelings of guilt in many who have become infected without being promiscuous. Sexual and physical contact should be avoided when the virus is active.

Abdominal Pain

There are all sorts of possible explanations for this, especially as there are so many different organs in the compact area of the pelvis. Many women notice a sharp pain low in the abdomen in the middle of a menstrual cycle which can be felt for five minutes or linger for two days. This is caused by ovulation, as a result of abdominal pressure from the enlargement of the ovary and follicle. Such enlargement often occurs during the normal course of ovulation and many women are told they have a cyst 'as big as an orange' on their ovaries. Generally the ovary shrinks back to its smaller size within a couple of weeks – so women should ask for several consecutive examinations over the course of a month to determine whether they truly do have a cyst.

Gas in the intestines can sometimes result in considerable discomfort, as can constipation. Pelvic inflammatory disease, and inflammation of the uterus and ovaries, can also cause lower abdominal pain, as can flu viruses, appendicitis, gall-bladder problems and urinary-tract infection. Prolonged or severe pain can be the result of tubal pregnancy. This is an emergency and needs immediate attention.

Crabs

Most women who have crabs know from the incessant itching that something is awry. The eggs take from seven to nine days to hatch and each crab busily lays three eggs a day.

Crabs are easily transmitted not only by sexual contact but by sitting on the same couch, using the same toilet, or by sharing a bed with someone who has them.

To 3 fl oz (90 ml) olive oil add 10 drops each of rosemary oil and lavender oil, 12 drops eucalyptus oil and 13 drops geranium oil. Saturate the area infested (usually the pubic area although they can survive in any hairy part of the body) with the oil and cover with close-fitting plastic pants or wrap the area in cling film. Leave on for two hours. Remove over the toilet and shampoo out. Comb through the hair with a finely toothed comb to remove any eggs. Repeat the treatment after three days, and again after a further three days.

Breast Lumps

Self-examination of the breasts after each menstruation is a vital prerequisite for discovering breast cysts and any more serious problems. Breast cysts are extraordinarily common and are almost always benign. Over 30 per cent of all women have these benign, fibrous, glandular growths. Cysts move easily under the fingers and are hard and round, tending to become larger and more tender just before menstruation. Women with a cyst often have increased fibrous tissue in their breasts because the cyst's lining and the adjacent connective tissue tend to be more fibrous. They are more common in women on the Pill or other hormones.

Caffeine has a stiffening effect on fibrous and connective tissues – so no coffee and chocolate whatsoever! Regular skin brushing helps, as does the poultice on page 115, and cleansing the lymphatic system (see Chapter 3).

Pre-orgasmic Problems

There is no real clinical or research experience that proves that pelvic congestion can lead to serious health problems. During the sexual excitement phase of a woman's sexual response the uterus, vagina, clitoris and vulva fill with blood and swell until they reach a state of vasocongestion, swelling which often causes tension and pressure. The medical profession insist that this can only be relieved by orgasm but in fact exercise, cold showers and the passage of time will do the same thing – though not as pleasurably!

So let's scotch the myth that women must have an orgasm in order to be healthy and that if they don't something is wrong.

But if it is orgasms you want, bear in mind that the single most common cause for a woman failing to reach orgasm is inadequate stimulation, but there are other possibilities – underdevelopment of the endocrine and nervous systems, diabetes, fear or ignorance, or immaturity of the female or male genitalia. Obvious emotional causes should be approached through counselling and will require co-operation from both partners.

Physical causes will need to be looked at individually. The following formula may help.

Equal parts of:

sarsaparilla
saw palmetto
damiana
liquorice
cinnamon
prickly ash bark

Take two size 'O' capsules of the finely powdered herbs with each meal daily for six months only. If you have high blood pressure leave out the liquorice, substituting the same amount of ginger.

Damiana has a marked effect on the sexual system, while prickly ash bark will stimulate the blood circulation. Cinnamon is warming; sarsaparilla is an excellent blood-purifier; saw palmetto is rich in natural hormones; and liquorice will bolster the adrenal glands and help to counteract stress.

Sexual Desire

ANAPHRODISIACS

A lot of people treat the subject of substances that dampen sexual desire as a joke. But there are many reasons why a woman may want to dampen her sexual fires: going through a prolonged healing crisis where the body needs plenty of rest; practising natural birth control which requires a couple only to make love during the infertile phases; choosing to live alone and remain celibate.

Avoid garlic, spices, meat, eggs, onion, salt, peppermint, too much alcohol, and stimulating books and television programmes, and take the following herbal formulation:

2 parts white willow
1 part scullcap
1 part white waterlily
1 part hops
1 part marjoram

Make into a tincture and take 2 teaspoons before each meal.

APHRODISIACS

Most traditional aphrodisiacs work by increasing your inclination, which is only half of the equation. The other half is, of course, the right partner, but if you want to try a little extra help take a massage of rose oil, sandalwood oil, jasmine oil or ylang-ylang oil. Rose oil is especially good for cleansing and regulating the gynaecological organs.

Abortion

Herbs like tansy and pennyroyal induce abortion, but a herbal abortion is even more traumatic for the body than a medical one and is therefore absolutely inadvisable. If you have already had an abortion, make plentiful use of such herbs as blessed thistle, raspberry, blue vervain and nettles to help restore the glandular system and bring the womb back to normal.

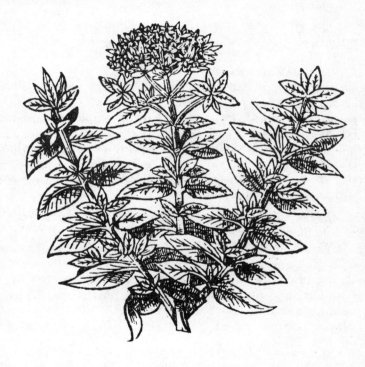

Appendix

Suppliers

HERBS, PREPARATIONS, ETC.

Stoke Lacy Herb Garden, Nr Bromyard, Herefordshire. Tel 043278 232

Iden Croft Herbs, Frittenden Road, Staplehurst, Kent. Tel 0580 891432

Oak Cottage Herb Farm, Nesscliffe, Nr Shrewsbury, Shropshire. Tel 074381 262

Herbs from the Hoo, 46 Church Street, Buckden, Cambridgeshire. Tel 0480 810818

Good-quality dried herbs are available by mail order and for personal callers from:

Neal's Yard Apothecary, 2 Neal's Yard, Covent Garden, London WC2. Tel 01-371 7662

Baldwins, 173 Walworth Road, London SE17. Tel 01-703 5550

Gerard House, 736 Christchurch Road, Boscombe, Bournemouth, Hampshire. Tel 0202 35352

D. Napier & Sons, 17–18 Bristol Place, Edinburgh, Scotland. Tel 031-225 5542

This company will generally not supply herbs in lesser amounts than 1 kg:

Brome & Schimmer, Great Bridge Road Estate, Romsey, Hampshire SO5 0HR. Tel 0794 515595

A wide selection of powdered herbs is available from:

Kitty Campion, The Natural Health and Iridology Centre, 19 Park Terrace, Tunstall, Stoke-on-Trent, Staffordshire ST6 6PB. Tel 0782 819855

An excellent range of essential oils is available in individual dropper bottles from:
Butterbur & Sage Ltd, PO Box 41, Southall, Middlesex, UB1 3BZ

Excellent-quality vitamins and minerals including amino-acids are available from:
Nature's Best, PO Box 1, Tunbridge Wells, Kent TN2 3EQ. Tel 0892 34143

This company manufactures high-quality nutritional supplements:
G. R. Lane, Sissons Road, Gloucester. Tel 0452 24012

Rescue Remedy is available from:
The Doctor Edward Bach Centre, Mount Vernon, Sotwell, Wallingford, Oxfordshire OX10 0PX.

Organic wines are available from:
Organic Wines and West Heath Wine, West Heath, Pirbright, Surrey GU24 0QE. Tel 04867 6464

Organic vegetables are available from growers who are members of:
The Soil Association, 86/88 Colston Street, Bristol BS1 5BB. Tel 0272 290667

Superdophilus and aloe vera juice are both available from:
G & G Food Supplies, 51 Railway Approach, East Grindstead, West Sussex RH19 1BT. Tel 0342 23016

Both should be kept refrigerated once opened. The prevention or maintenance dose of Superdophilus is 0.5 g once daily (two weeks on, one week off) for a minimum of six months. The therapeutic dose is 5–10 g a day for up to eight days, followed by the prevention or maintenance dosage. All doses should be taken in 8 fl oz (230 ml) lukewarm water between meals and as far away from anything containing sugar as possible.

Probion is available from:
Natural Flow, Burwash Common, East Sussex. Tel 0435 882482

Probion comes in bottles of 180 tablets. The normal therapeutic course is two tablets chewed or swallowed with food twice daily.

The tablets can be taken orally or used as vaginal or anal suppositories. The transient bacteria in Probion provide the greatest benefit when taken over a period of two to four months. Anyone with a skin condition will need to take Probion for a minimum of five months and possibly even a year before they see a sudden dramatic improvement, whereas acute holiday diarrhoea may be checked by 5–10 tablets three times daily for a few days only.

EQUIPMENT
Enema and douche kits and natural-bristle skin brushes as well as gelatin capsules are available from:
Kitty Campion, The Natural Health and Iridology Centre, 19 Park Terrace, Tunstall, Stoke-on-Trent, Staffordshire ST6 6PB. Tel 0782 819855

Ionizers are available from:
South Eastern Ionizer Centre, Machico House, Primrose Hill, Fairlight, East Sussex

Mini-trampolines at reasonable prices are available by mail order from:
Mangoletri Trampolines, 205 Drayton Bridge Road, Ealing, London W13 0JH

Training to be a Medical Herbalist

Kitty Campion is a director of the School of Natural Healing, UK, together with Jill Davies. The school was founded over half a century ago in Utah, USA by Dr Christopher, America's foremost wholistic herbalist. It trains students to be herbal practitioners, awarding the advanced American qualification of Master Herbalist, but it also offers an introductory course in herbal and diet healing to interested amateurs. This course leads to the qualification of Herbal Diploma, which is designed to equip those working in the retail food business, but is definitely *not* a qualification to practise. For details on the HD and MH courses and a list of practitioners holding the qualification of MH nationwide write to Kitty Campion.

An alternative medical course which is not so wholistic but which is nevertheless sound is available from the National Institute of Medical Herbalists, 41 Hatherley Road, Winchester, Hampshire SO22 6RR. This school also supplies a list of practitioners holding the qualification of NIMH.

QUALIFICATIONS MATTER
As interest in natural medicine grows, an astonishing number of self-styled healers are jumping on the bandwagon, and because most of them are not trained in diagnostics they have an unfortunate tendency to treat the symptoms not the cause. This way they have some moderate successes. It is comparatively easy to remove the symptoms. It is quite another matter to get down to the cause by dint of patience and lots of detective work, and then to go on to educate patients as to how to heal themselves at this – the deepest – level.

A young girl came to see me who had lost 2 stone (12 kg) in two months because she felt so sick that she couldn't eat. She had extremely bad headaches and kept fainting. Her doctor dismissed her as a malingerer and was about to force her into hospital for intravenous feeding. Using iridology I discovered that a blow on the head had dislocated the cervical vertebrae in her neck and it was this that was causing all the pain. I referred her to an osteopath and she made an excellent and very rapid recovery.

Look for the qualifications mentioned above. As in every profession, the skill of medical herbalists will vary. Choose someone who fits into your lifestyle. You may go for the leather-thonged, red-shirted naturopath breathing fire and brimstone and carrot or you may prefer the white-coated, quieter approach. But whoever you choose look for and expect professionalism. I think the best way to make a choice is to talk to other patients working with the practitioner you have in mind. By their results shall you know them. If a patient has been going to see a practitioner for the last two years there is something wrong. This obviously means the disease is not being helped. Choose someone who specializes in one field only. The Jack-of-all-trades and master of none with a wall littered with weekend course certificates is no good to you. Be prepared to work with someone who will open-mindedly refer you onto another branch of naturopathy if necessary. Herbalism isn't the panacea for all ills.

222 A WOMAN'S HERBAL

Neither is acupuncture or osteopathy though some practitioners evidently believe so!

The only patients I tend to see for more than five or six visits are those with deeply entrenched diseases like multiple sclerosis or diabetes. I obviously love to see patients for a yearly health check-up on a preventative basis.

Other Useful Addresses

A register of well-trained iridologists throughout the country is available from:
The National Council & Register of Iridologists, 'Lacunga', 80 Portland Road, Bournemouth BH9 1NQ. Tel 0202 529793

For information about the ongoing research into herbs as medicine join:
The British Herbal Medicine Association, Lane House, Cowling, Keighley, West Yorkshire BD22 0LX

At the time of writing, the Department of Health and Security is threatening the survival of more than 1,000 natural medicines. If you feel as strongly as I do that the DHSS should not be allowed to do this please join the Natural Medicine Society. Ordinary membership currently costs £5.
Natural Medicine Society, Edith Lewis House, Back Lane, Ilkeston, Derby DE7 8ET

For help with post-natal illness contact:
The Association of Post-natal Illness, 7 Gowan Avenue, Fulham, London SW6

Pilates technique, a well-worked-out unique system of body realignment is available on personal application to:
Alan Herdman, Pilates Technique, 17 Homer Row, London W1. Tel 01-723 9953
For cystitis sufferers support and advice is available from:
U&I Club, 9E Compton Road, London N1. Tel 01-359 0403

Ingredients Which Can Cause Allergic Reactions

Some people are allergic even to water, and everything and anything can cause an allergic reaction in someone. I have known women to react to innocuous ingredients like lanolin, henna, glycerine and certain essential oils, all ingredients which have been used safely and effectively by most people for thousands of years. If the ingredients listed in this book are not used properly, if they are taken in excess, used for too long a time, used stale when it has specifically stated that they should be fresh, or taken internally when recommended for external use, they may cause an allergic reaction. Patch-testing as described on page 80 is advisable for the external use of any ingredient you feel may be suspect. The following list of herbs and other cosmetic aids can sometimes cause allergic reactions. These are rare but nevertheless worth noting.

agrimony, arrowroot, benzoin tincture, birch sap, birch bark, buttercup, camphor, camomile, coconut butter, cornstarch, cowslips, daisy, glycerine, golden-seal, greater celandine, henna, honeysuckle, hops, horseradish, ivy, lanolin, stale lime blossom, linseed oil, lovage, mistletoe berries, mugwort, mustard, myrrh tincture, nasturtium, nettles, orris-root, pansy, paw-paw, penny-royal, pineapple, pine-needles, plantain, primrose, quince seed, rue, Solomon's-seal, southernwood, strawberries, sulphonated castor oil, tansy, white willow bark, wormwood, violet leaves, yellow sandalwood

Essential oils of: basil, bay, bergamot, clary sage, neroli, penny-royal, peppermint, sage, spearmint

References

CHAPTER 1

Williams, Roger, *Nutrition Against Disease*, New York, Pitman, 1971.

Williams, Roger, *Biochemical Individuality*, Austin and London, 1979.

Campion, Kitty, *Kitty Campion's Handbook of Herbal Health*, Sphere, 1985.

Campion, Kitty, *Kitty Campion's Vegetarian Encyclopaedia*, Century Hutchinson, 1986.

CHAPTER 3
Hirayama, T., 'Passive smoking and lung cancer, a nasal sinus, cancer, brain tumour and ischemic heart disease in', *Proceedings of the Fifth World Conference on Smoking and Health*, 1985, Vol. 1: 137–41.
Garland, C., 'Effects of passive smoking on ischemic heart disease mortality in non-smokers', *The American Journal of Epidemiology*, 1985, 121: 645–50.
Freler, R., 'Independence of mechanisms that control bacterial colonisation of large intestine', *Microecology and Therapy*, 1983, Vol. 13: 55–60.
Grant, Doris & Joice, Jean, *Food Combining for Health*, Wellingborough, Thorsons, 1984.

CHAPTER 5
Phillips, Roger, *Wild Flowers of Britain*, Pan Books Limited, 1977.

CHAPTER 9
Bairacli-Levy, Juliette de, *Nature's Children*, Schocken Books, New York, 1971.

CHAPTER 11
Airola, Paavo, 'Menopause: a Dreadful Affliction or Glorious Experience – Nutritional and Other Biological Solutions to Menopausal Problems, Oestrogen Therapy and Premature Ageing', *Let's Live Magazine*, July 1976.

Botanical Index

Aconite *Aconitum Napellus*
Agrimony *Agrimonia Enpatoria*
Alfalfa *Medicago Sativa*
Allspice *Pimento Officinalis*
Almond *Amygdalus Communis*
Aloe *Aloe Vera*
Angelica *Angelica Archangelica*
Anise *Pimpinella Anisum*
Aniseed *Pimpinella Anisum*
Arnica *Arnica Montana*
Arrow Root *Maranta Arundinaceae*
Artichoke *Cynara Scolymus*
Ash *Fraxinus Excelsior*
Autumn Crocus *Colchicum Autumnale*

Balm, Lemon *Melissa Officinalis*
Balm of Gilead *Populus Gileadensis*
Barley *Hordeum Distichon*

Basil *Ocimum Basilicum*
Bay Laurel *Laurel Nobilis*
Bayberry *Myrica Cerifera*
Bearberry *Arctostaphylos Uva-ursi*
Belladonna *Atropa Belladonna*
Benzoin *Styrax Benzoin*
Bergamot *Monarda Didyma*
Beth Root *Trillium Pendulum*
(Wood) Betony *Stachys Betonica*
Bilberry *Vaccinium Myrtillus*
Birch *Betula Alba*
Black Cohosh *Cimicifuga Racemosa*
Black Horehound *Ballota Nigra*
Black Walnut *Juglans Nigra*
Blessed Thistle *Cnicus Benedictus*
Blue Cohosh *Caulophyllum Thalictroides*
Blue Flag *Iris Versicolor*
Blue Rue *Ruta Graveolens*

Boneset *Eupatorium Perfoliatum*
Brooklime *Veronica Beccabunga*
Borage *Borago Officinalis*
Bramble *Rubus Fructicosus*
Broom *Cytisus Scoparius*
Buchu *Barosma Betulina*
Buckwheat *Fagopyrum Esculentum*
Buckthorn *Rhamnus Cathartica*
Burdock *Arctium Lappa*
Butterbur *Petasites Vulgaris*
Buttercup *Ranunculus Bulbosus*
(White) Bryony *Bryonia Dioica*

Calamus *Acorus Calumus*
Camphor *Cinnamonum Camphora*
Cape Aloes *Aloe Ferox*
Castor Oil Plant *Ricinus Communis*

Caraway *Carum Carvi*
Carrot (Wild) *Daucus Corota*
Cascara Sagrada *Rhamnus Purshianus*
Castor Oil *Ricinus Communis*
Catnip *Nepeta Cataria*
Cayenne *Capsicum Minimum*
(Greater) Celandine *Chelidonium Majus*
Celery *Apium Graveolens*
Matricaria *Chamomilla*
Common *Anthemis Nobilis*
Chamomile German
Chaparral *Larrea Divaricata Cav*
Chasteberries *Agnus Castus*
(Horse) Chestnut *Aesculus Hippocastanum*
Chevril *Anthriscus Cerefolium*
Chickweed *Stellaria Media*

Chicory *Cichorium*
Intybus
Chive *Allium*
Sclcenoprasum
(Sweet) Cicely
Myrrhis
Odorata
Cinnamon
Cinnamonum
Zeylanicum
Clary Sage *Salvia*
Horminoides
Cleavers *Galium*
Aparine
Clove *Eugenia*
Caryophyllata
(Red) Clover
Trifolium
Pratense
Coltsfoot *Tussilaga*
Farfara
Comfrey
Symphytum
Officinale
Cornflower
Centaurea
Cyanus
Cornsilk *Zea Mays*
Couch Grass
Agropyrum
Repens
Cowslip *Primula*
Veris
Cramp Bark
Viburnum
Opulus
Cranberry
Vaccinum
Macrocarpon
Cucumber
Cucumis
Sativa
(Red) Currant
Ribes
Rubrum

Daisy *Bellis*
Perennis
Damiana *Damiana*
Aphrodisiaca
Dandelion
Taraxacum
Officinale

Dill *Anethum*
Graveolens
(Yellow) Dock
Rumex
Crispus
Dulse *Fucus*
Vesiculosis

Echinacea
Echinacea
Angustifolia
Elder (Berry)
Sambucus Nigra
Elecampagne *Inula*
Helenium
(Slippery) Elm
Ulmus
Fulva
Eucalyptus
Eucalyptus
Globulus
(Evening) Primrose
Oenothera
Biennis
Eyebright
Euphrasia
Officinalis

Fennel *Foeniculum*
Vulgare
Fenugreek
Trigonella
Foenum –
Graecum
Feverfew
Chrysanthemum
Parthenium
Figwort (Knotted)
Scrophularia
Nodosa
Flax *Linum*
Usitatissimum
Foxglove *Digitalis*
Purpurea
Fumitory *Fumaria*
Officinalis

Garlic *Allium*
Sativum
Gentian *Gentiana*
(Yellow) Gentian
Gentiana Lutca
Geranium

Geranium
Maculatum
Ginger (Root)
Zingiber
Officinale
Ginseng
Asiatic: *Panax*
Ginseng
Siberian:
Eleutherococcus
Senticosus
Gipsy Weed
Lycopus
Europaeus
Goat's Rue *Galega*
Officinalis
Goldenseal
Hydrastis
Canadensis
Gotu Kola
Hydrocotyle
Asiatica
Grapes (Oregan
Grape
Root) *Berberis*
Aquifolium
Gravel Root
Eupatorium
Purpureum
Grindelia *Grindelia*
Camporium
Grindelia
Cuneifolia
Grindelia
Squarrosa
Groundsel *Senecio*
Viscosus

Hawthorn
Crataegus
Monogyna
Heartsease *Viola*
Tricolor
Heather *Calluna*
Vulgaris
(Red) Hibiscus
Rosa –
Sinensis
(False) Hellebore
Adonis
Autumnalis
Hemlock *Conium*
Maculatum

Henna *Lawsonia*
Alba
Holly *Ilex*
Aquifolium
Honeysuckle
Lonicera
Caprifolium
Hops *Humulus*
Lupulus
Horehound
Marrubium
Vulgare
Horse Radish
Cochlearia
Armoracia
Horsetail
Equisetum
Houseleek
Sempervivum
Tectorum
Hydrangea (Root)
Hydrangea
Arborescens
Hyssop *Hyssopus*
Officinalis

Ipecac *Cephaelis*
Ipecacuanha
Iris *Iris Versicolor*
(Ground) Ivy
Glechoma
Hederacea

Jasmine (General)
Jasminum
Juniper *Juniperus*
Communis

Kava Kava *Piper*
Methysticum
Kelp *Fucus*
Vesiculosus

Lady's Mantle
Alchemilla
Vulgaris
Lady's Slipper
Cypripedium
Pubescens
Lavender *Santolina*
Cotton Lavender
Chamaecy
Parissus

English Lavender
  Lavandula Vera
Lemon Citrus
  Limonum
Lemon Balm
  Melissa
  Officinalis
Lettuce Lactuca
  Virosa
(White Water) Lily
  Nymphaea
  Odorata
Lime Citrus Acida
Linseed (Flax)
  Linum
  Usitatissimum
Liquorice
  Glycyrrhiza
  Glabra
Lobelia Lobelia
  Inflata
(Purple) Loosestrife
  Lythrum
  Salicaria
Lovage Levisticum
  Officinale
Lungwort Sticta
  Pulmonaria
Lupin
  Leguminosae

Malefern
  Dryopteris
  Felix-mas
Mandrake Atropa
  Mandragora
Marigold
  Calendula
  Officinalis
Marjoram
  Sweet Origanum
  Marjorana
  Wild Origanum
  Vulgare
Meadowsweet
  Filipendula
  Ulmaria
Mimosa Mimosa
  Fragifolia
(Spear) Mint
  Mentha
  Viridis
Mistletoe Viscum

Album
(Icelandic) Moss
  Cetraria
  Islandica
(Irish) Moss
  Chondrus
  Crispus
Sphagnum Moss
  Sphagnum
  Cymbifolium
Motherwort
  Leonurus
  Cardiaca
Mugwort
  Artemisia
  Vulgaris
Mullein
  Verbascum
  Thapsus
Mustard
  Black Brassica
  Nigra
  White Brassica
  Alba
Myrrh
  Commiphora
  Myrrha

Nasturtium
  Tropaeolum
  Majus
Neroli (Orange)
  Citrus
  Aurantium
Nettles Urticaceae
Nutmeg Myristica
  Fragrans

Oak Lavercus
  Robur
Oats Avena Sativa
Olive Olea
  Europaea
Onion Allium Cepa
Orange
  Bitter Citrus
  Vulgaris
  Sweet Citrus
  Aurantium
(Wild) Orchid
  Orchid
  Masculata
Oregon Grape

Root
  Berberis
  Aquifolium
Origanum Vulgare
  Aureum
Orris Root Iris
  Florentina

Pansy Viola
  Tricolor
Parsley
  Petroselinum
  Sativum
Passion Flower
  Anemone
  Pusatilla
Peach Prunus
  Persica
Pellitory of the
  Wall
  Parietaria
  Officinalis
Penny Royal
  Mentha
  Pulegium
Peppermint
  Mentha
  Piperita
Periwinkle
  (Greater)
  Vinca Major
Pilewort
  Ranunculus
  Ficaria
Pine Pinaceae
Plantain Plantago
  Major
Pleurisy Root
  Asclepias
  Tuberose
Poke Root
  Phytolacca
  Decandra
Pomegranate
  Punica
  Granatum
Prickly Ash
  Xanthoxylum
  Americanum
Primrose Primula
  Vulgaris
Privet Liqustrum
  Vulgare

Psyllium Plantago
  Psyllium
Pulsatilla Anemone
  Pulsatilla
Purslane
  Green Portulaca
  Oleracea
  Golden
  Portulaca
  Sativa

Quassia (Bark)
  Picraena Excelsa
Quince Pyrus
  Cydonia

Raspberry Rubus
  Idaeus
Rest-Harrow
  Ononis
  Arvensis
(Turkey) Rhubarb
  Rheum
  Palmatum
Rose Roseceae
Rosehip Rosa
  Canina
Rosemary
  Rosemarinus
  Officinalis
Rue Ruta
  Graveolens

Sage Salvia
  Officinalis
(Yellow)
  Sandalwood
  Santalum Album
Sassafras Sassafras
  Officinale
Savory
  Summer Satureia
  Hortensis
  Winter Satureia
  Montano
Saw Palmetto
  Sarenoa
  Serrulata
Scabious Field
  Scabiosa
  Arvensis
Scullcap
  (Virquinian)

Scullcap – *Cont.*
Scutellaria
Lateriflora
Seaweed (General)
Fucus Vesiculosis
Self-heal *Prunella*
Vulgaris
Senna *Cassia*
Acutifolia
Shepherd's Purse
Capsella
Bursa-Pastoris
Soap Wort
Saponaria
Officinalis
Solomon's
Seal
Polygonatum
Multiflorum
Sorrel
French *Rumex*
Scatatus
Garden *Rumex*
Acetosa
Southernwood
Field
Artemisia
Campestria
Speedwell
Common
Veronica

Officinalis
Squaw Vine
Mitchella
Repens
Squill *Urginea*
Scilla
St John's Wort
Hypericum
Perforatum
Stillingia *Stillingia*
Sylvatica
Stone Root
Collinsonia
Canadensis
Strawberry
Fragaria
Vesca
Sunflower
Helianthus
Annvus

Tansy *Tanacetum*
Vulgare
Thuja *Thuja*
Occidentalis
Thyme
Garden *Thymus*
Vulgaris
Wild *Thymus*
Serpyllum

Toad Flax *Linaria*
Vulgaris
Tobacco *Nicotiana*
Tabacum
Tormentil
Potentilla
Tormentilla
Tumeric *Curcuma*
Longa

(False) Unicorn
Chamaelirium
Luteum
(True) Unicorn
Aletris
Farinosa
Uva-Ursi
Arctostaphylos
Uva-Ursi

Valerian *Valeriana*
Officinalis
Vervain (Blue)
Verbena
Officinalis
Vine (General)
Vitis
Vinifera
Violet (Sweet)

Viola
Odorata

Watercress
Nasturtium
Officinale
(White) Willow
Salix
Alba
(Rosebay)
Willow-Herb
Epilobium
Angustifolium
Winter Green
Gaultheria
Procumbens
Witch Hazel
Hamamelis
Virginiana
Woodruff *Asperula*
Odorata
Wormwood
(Common)
Artemisia
Absinthium
(Wild) Yam
Dioscorea
Villosa

Yarrow *Achillea*
Millefolium

Index